ACTIVE BIRTH

P9-DXZ-608

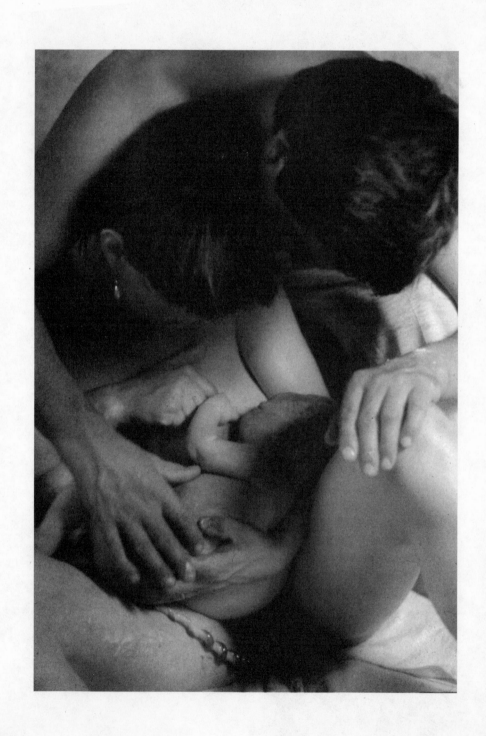

ACTIVE BIRTH
The New Approach to Giving Birth Naturally

REVISED EDITION

Janet Balaskas

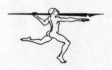

THE HARVARD COMMON PRESS
Harvard and Boston, Massachusetts

The Harvard Common Press
535 Albany Street
Boston, Massachusetts 02118

First edition published in 1983 by Unwin Paperbacks, London, as
Active Birth.

Second edition published in 1991 by Thorsons, an imprint of Grafton
Books, London, as *New Active Birth: A Concise Guide to Natural
Childbirth*.

This U.S. edition published in 1992 by The Harvard Common Press.

Printed in the United States of America.

Library of Congress Cataloging-in-Publication Data

Balaskas, Janet.
   Active birth : the new approach to giving birth naturally / by
Janet Balaskas ; foreword by Sheila Kitzinger ; introduction by
Michel Odent. — Rev. ed.
     p.   cm.
   Includes bibliographical references (p.   ) and index.
                  ISBN 1-55832-038-5
   1. Active childbirth.   2. Exercise for women.   I. Title.
RG662.B35   1992
618.4—dc20   91-32334

Photographs by Anthea Sieveking
Illustrations by Lucy Su and Laura McKechnie
Cover design by Jackie Schuman

10 9 8 7 6 5 4

Contents

Contents

Acknowledgments

First I would like to thank all of the mothers and their families whose experiences fill the pages of this book.

Thanks also to those who helped to produce it, especially Anthea Sieveking for the photographs, Linda Ziedrich for editing the U.S. edition, Penny Simkin for her thoughtful editorial suggestions, and the staff at the Harvard Common Press. And thanks to Sheila Kitzinger for introducing me to the Harvard Common Press, and to Jennifer Starisky, senior midwife at the Garden Hospital, for compiling the hospital's 1990 statistics especially for this book.

I am very grateful to my colleagues Lolly Stirk and Yvonne Moore for helping to establish the Active Birth Teachers Training Course; to Yehudi Gordon, Michel Odent, and midwives everywhere for their pioneering work; as well as yoga teachers Mina Semyon, Mary Stuart, and Lolly and John Stirk for their inspiration.

Profound thanks to Carole Eliott for her guidance and to her husband Norman Stannard for his healing energy. Most of all I would like to thank my four children for helping me discover the great joy of giving birth and being a mother and my husband Keith Brainin for his loving support and encouragement.

Foreword

Here is an important voice in childbirth. Janet Balaskas is speaking to those women who want to grow in self-awareness and to use their bodies actively in labor. In her childbirth classes Janet Balaskas stands for activity rather than passivity, for movement rather than immobilization, and for a woman's right to choose whatever position she finds comfortable throughout labor and delivery.

The teaching in this book is revolutionary. Yet it is age-old. All over the world and throughout recorded history women have chosen upright positions to give birth, and it is only we in the West who have had the extraordinary notion that a woman should lie on her back with her legs in the air to deliver a baby.

But to get women upright is to do much more than help them find a comfortable posture. It is to turn them from passive patients into active birth-givers. It is to challenge the whole obstetric view of birth in Western society. This is based on the assumption that childbirth is a medical event that should be conducted in an intensive-care setting. The whole pregnancy is seen as a pathological condition terminated only by delivery. The modern high-tech obstetrician actively manages labor with all the technology of ultrasound, continuous electronic monitoring, and intravenous oxytocin drip. Many obstetricians have never had the opportunity to see a truly natural birth. To turn the process of bringing new life into the world into one in which a woman becomes simply the body on the delivery table rather than an active birth-giver is a degradation of the mother's role in childbirth.

We are now beginning to discover the sometimes long-term destructive effects on the relationship between a mother and her baby, and on the family, of treating women as if they were merely containers to be relieved of their contents, and of concentrating attention on a bag of muscle and a birth canal, instead of relating to and caring for the person of whom the uterus and the vagina are a part.

Bonding is a fashionable term today. In many hospitals special time is devoted for bonding, and there must be few midwives and obstetricians who would not claim that they consider bonding important. But everything that happens after delivery is the outcome of what has gone before. Bonding is either spontaneous and easy, or made virtually impossible by the atmosphere at delivery and by the care a woman is given as a *person*, not merely a "para 1," an elderly primigravida, a maternal pelvis, a contracting uterus, or a dilating cervix.

The way we give birth is important to all of us because it has a great deal to do with the kind of society we want to live in, the significance of the coming to birth of a new person and a new family.

When we hand over responsibility for choosing between alternatives on the basis of what we believe to be right, we hand over responsibility for the quality of the society we, and our children, must live in.

Sheila Kitzinger

Preface

My first daughter, Nina, was born in 1970. I attended preparation classes and was hoping for a natural birth. I was active until strong labor began, and then I lay passively in bed, semireclining, for the last three hours. Fortunately there were no complications, and I managed, with enormous effort and the help of an unnecessary episiotomy, to give birth to her spontaneously.

I discovered active childbirth during the birth of my second daughter, Kim. During this pregnancy I had taken up yoga and enjoyed practicing the yoga postures, finding some of them particularly beneficial as the pregnancy advanced. A study of the history of childbirth revealed how some of the yoga postures, especially squatting, are similar to birth positions used throughout the ages. An anatomical study of the female pelvis clarified that these postures relaxed and "opened" the pelvic canal and were ideal movements to adopt when trying to evacuate its contents.

Consequently, when it came to labor, I began by following the usual instructions given in prenatal classes and made myself comfortable in the semireclining position, focusing on some breathing techniques. Progress was slow, and while the breathing techniques kept me calm and centered, they seemed to distract me from the labor. Eventually I decided to get up and try some of the positions I had practiced during pregnancy. The change in progress was dramatic, and it dawned on me, for the first time, that it is necessary for a woman to move and to be in harmony with gravity in order to help her body to open up in labor. I realized then that squatting, and its variations, is the logical position for any woman to adopt while giving birth and is the most important position to practice during pregnancy. I resolved then and there to improve my squatting before my next labor.

During my son Iasonas's birth I kept active—walking, squatting, and kneeling—and gave birth to him on all fours. It was a marvelous experience. I had an entirely new sense of control and knew instinctively what to do. I was up within hours of the birth and felt none of the aches and pains I had for a week or two after my previous births, despite the fact that he was almost a 10-pound baby. I was astonished how fit and well I felt after the birth, and I suffered no exhaustion or depression in the following months.

In 1988 number four was born, also at home. Theo weighed in at 11 pounds, and this time I had a portable water birth pool, designed by my husband Keith, in our bedroom. Labor was intense, and as soon as I reached 5 centimeters dilation I entered the pool. The buoyancy of the water made it much easier for me to relax. I was encouraged to let myself go without any inhibitions, and I remember making a tremendous amount of noise and reaching full dilation very quickly.

Michel Odent, who was in attendance, suggested that I leave the pool for the actual birth. Given Theo's size, we decided that I needed the help of gravity to get him born, so I used the supported standing squat position. He was born in two contractions despite his size, miraculously without a tear. The medical establishment would certainly have considered me "high risk." I was 42 and Rh-negative, and had had surgery on the uterus three years previously. These were the very reasons that I wanted to stay at home, where conditions for a normal birth were optimal.

My own birth experiences are not unusual. Since 1978 I have been teaching yoga to pregnant women, and more than 80 percent of them have succeeded in giving birth naturally and actively to their babies. Most of them have had no previous experience of yoga, and their ages have ranged from 19 to 49. It has been a joy to observe how readily their bodies have responded to the yoga. As their flexibility has improved, their health and happiness have increased. At the end of pregnancy most of them have been in touch with their birthing and motherly instincts and have been able to approach birth with confidence. The experiences of these women have added to my personal conviction and won support from their midwives, doctors, and obstetricians.

Many women enjoy the benefits of yoga so much that they are back in the mother and baby exercise sessions two to three weeks after birth. This is so not only in the case of the mothers who have had normal, problem-free births, but sometimes also for those who have needed the help of forceps or cesarean section.

Over the years I have seen that keeping active during labor and adopting natural, upright or crouching birth positions is the safest, most enjoyable, most economical and sensible way for the majority of women to give birth. There is no disruption of the normal physiology of labor, no interference with the hormonal balance. Postnatal depression is rare, and problems with breastfeeding and mothering are less likely.

The majority of labors—managed well—should be uncomplicated. No special equipment is needed, and the birth can take place in the simplest environment or in the most sophisticated hospital delivery room. Active birth is natural and instinctive. It is the way a woman, left to her own devices, will behave during labor. In preparing a woman for an active birth, my aim is to help her get in touch with her own birth-giving instinct.

Giving birth is essentially a natural bodily function that occurs quite spontaneously and involuntarily at the end of pregnancy. It is part of a continuous evolution that begins with lovemaking and conception and ends in the growing independence of the child from his or her mother during the first few years of life. The whole process of conceiving a baby, being pregnant, giving birth, and mothering is part of the sexual and spiritual life of a woman, and is basically rooted in the natural and undisturbed unfolding of a series of physiological events. The best way in which a woman entering into motherhood can prepare herself is by working on her own body.

The yoga exercises I recommend are not unnatural movements imposed upon the body. On the contrary, they are instinctive and simple movements we could all make with ease. I teach a kind of physical "remembering" rather than a system of exercise. In fact, many of the exercises in this book came from my observations of the movements made by my children when they were very young. By watching them, I realized how stiff, as adults, we have become; how we have lost contact with the range of movement nature intended us to have. A toddler will squat with ease for a long time, feet flat on the ground, back straight, and rise up from this position when she walks.

It is well known that the more civilized we become the more we forget our natural habits. Today we are able to ensure a reliable medical backup, in the event of complications, for all women giving birth, and the mortality rate has been improved by the lifesaving techniques of modern obstetrics. As I have seen all too often in my practice, however, the widespread use of routine obstetric technology, inappropriately applied to normal labor, disturbs the natural birth process and causes many of the problems it was designed to prevent. In some hospitals, birth has become an abdominal or vaginal extraction conducted as if on a conveyor belt. The result is that most women are completely out of touch with their own instinctive ability to give birth, and practitioners are losing their intuitive skills as they depend more on technology. Many women have never seen a birth or even held a baby by the time they enter motherhood. The natural skills of giving birth and mothering are no longer handed down from woman to woman, generation to generation.

We can regain a link with our female heritage by re-educating our bodies in the habits, movements, and postures that are instinctive to the childbearing woman. In pregnancy, when the whole tendency of the body is towards health and vitality, a woman has a unique opportunity to work on herself.

The main concern of this book is normal birth and the common variations from the norm, which can usually be handled without obstetric intervention. Women who prepare for active birth and then find themselves faced with an unexpected complication or needing the help of pain-relieving drugs often find ways of successfully combining active birth with obstetric procedures.

I hope that this book will help to bring to light the simple common sense of childbirth, which has somehow been obscured in the advance of modern obstetrics, and will help women to rediscover their own inner resources for giving birth to their babies.

The Active Birth Movement

In the late 1970s a group of women in North London, recognizing the benefits of active birth, attempted to give birth in upright positions in a local hospital. Some of them met with success, encouraged to do so by an obstetrician, Yehudi Gordon, and his staff, while others encountered stubborn opposition. Conflict arose within the labor ward, which resulted in a "ban" being placed on active birth. Some mothers whose labors were imminent were extremely distressed, and they telephoned me to express their feelings. I felt responsible for introducing them to the concept of active birth. It seemed completely inappropriate for them to have to fight during their labors for the right to give birth instinctively.

Consequently the Active Birth Movement was founded in April 1982, and the Active Birth Manifesto was written.

The occasion was marked by a demonstration on Sunday, April 11, which we called the Birthrights Rally. Originally, we intended to hold a "squat-in" in the hospital foyer, but within a mere three weeks so many people were offering their support that we ended up on Hampstead Heath with a crowd of six thousand. The rally was a protest against hospitals that denied women the freedom to move about in labor and to give birth in upright, squatting, or kneeling positions, despite mounting evidence of the advantages.

Michel Odent, whose work in France helping women to give birth instinctively had been featured in the same year on British television, came to speak at the rally, along with Sheila Kitzinger, well-known author on childbirth, and other friends of active birth. The occasion was memorable, and it brought a change of attitude at the hospital, which has been able to accommodate women wanting active births ever since. Thankfully, the Active Birth Movement has not needed to stage another demonstration, as hospitals throughout London and further afield have gradually been adjusting to the climate of change.

Our main function since then has been educational, providing conferences, lectures, and workshops for parents and professionals, as well as training facilities for Active Birth teachers. We also provide a free advisory service from our London center (see "Resources").

Promising changes in maternity care and prenatal education have been happening simultaneously in many countries over the past decade. The Active Birth Movement is now international; it has branches in many parts of the world, many of which have had great success in stimulating change.

Although the Active Birth Movement as yet has no branch in the United States, the widespread and diverse North American alternative birth movement has long advocated mobility and upright positions in labor and childbirth. Beginning in the early 1980s, most American hospitals responded to consumer pressure by installing high-tech birthing chairs or the more popular and versatile "birthing beds." These beds can be configured to support laboring women in a wide variety of positions. Although birthing beds are standard equipment in most hospitals today, the frequency in which they are used to support women in upright positions varies from one hospital to another. In hospitals where the staff and patients rely heavily on epidural anesthesia, there is little interest in active birth. In other hospitals and in birth centers, the nurses, midwives, and doctors are comfortable with active birth and even promote it. Childbirth classes vary similarly. The principles of active birth will gradually be put into practice more widely as we learn more about the normal physiology of birth and about how many common practices can interfere with it. Change will happen slowly, however, unless women refuse to submit to conventional practices and begin to trust their own bodies.

The Active Birth Movement is run entirely by women like myself, who have rediscovered childbirth through their own experiences. They are women who have chosen to get off the obstetric delivery table and to give birth instinctively. Consequently they pass on what they have learned to others and through their work they are creating a new tradition of womanly wisdom, helping women everywhere to regain their autonomy as childbearers. Many have told me their birth stories, excerpts from which appear throughout chapters 6, 7, and 8.

It is to these women that I dedicate this book.

Intensive training courses in the Janet Balaskas method of preparation for active birth are held at the Active Birth Centre in London and are open to American childbirth educators and midwives. Audio and video cassettes on active birth are also available. For information contact the Active Birth Centre, 55 Dartmouth Park Road, London NW5 1SL.

Introduction

The concept of "active birth" is a milestone in the history of childbirth. Bringing together these two simple words is by itself a work of genius: *active birth* covers a huge scale of meanings, at different, complementary levels.

The first level might be described as muscular. When you just have a glimpse of some pictures of "active births" you notice that at the end of the labor, when the baby is coming, many mothers are vertical, hanging on to someone or something, or leaning forward on something, or in a supported squatting position, or kneeling.

At the second level you penetrate more deeply into the physiological process of childbirth. Childbirth is first a brain process. When a woman is giving birth by herself, the active part of her brain is the primitive part. It is this part that we have in common with all the mammals, the part that secretes the necessary hormones. A woman gives birth actively when she can secrete her own hormones, or, in other words, when she does not need synthetic hormones from a drip, or any other kind of medical intervention. The activity of the primitive part of the brain implies a reduction of inhibitions coming from the "new" brain, the neocortex. The factors that can disturb this brain process, this change in level of consciousness, such as noise, bright lights, and the presence of strangers, are not easily eliminated in the context of a modern obstetric unit. The ideal environment for an active birth ensures the mother privacy, semi-darkness, silence, and, at the same time, the proximity of an experienced person.

At the third level "active birth" refers to the attitude that society as a whole has towards childbirth. In our society childbirth is completely under the control and under the responsibility of medical institutions. Pregnant and laboring women are called "patients." Modern obstetric nurses, trained in obstetric units, are not simply mothers helping other mothers. When a newborn baby is not healthy, the medical institution is considered responsible. The concept of "active birth" has been intro-duced by women who want to take back the control and the responsibility of childbirth. They consider the medical institution as a resource to use in precise circumstances. What a provocative challenge at a time when the negative side effects of obstetrics are better and better known!

The day when Janet introduced the phrase "active birth" was possibly the most important one in the history of childbirth in Europe since the day when the French doctor Mauriceau took control of childbirth as he placed the laboring woman on her back.

Michel Odent

1 | What Is an Active Birth?

DURING THE RAPID DEVELOPMENT OF MODERN OBSTET-rics in the past three hundred years, women have lost touch with their power as birth-givers. We have almost forgotten how a natural physiological birth unfolds.

An active birth is nothing new. It is simply a convenient way of describing normal labor and birth and the way that a woman behaves when she is following her own instincts and the physiological logic of her body. It is a way of saying that she herself controls her body while giving birth, rather than being the passive recipient of a birth that is managed by her attendants.

By deciding to have an active birth you will be reclaiming your fundamental power as a birth-giver, a mother, and a woman. You will also be giving your baby the best possible start in life and a safe transition from the womb to the world. Should an unusual difficulty or complication arise, you will be free to make use of the safety net of modern obstetric care, knowing that you have done your very best and also knowing that this is your choice and that the intervention was really necessary. In this way, even the most difficult birth can be a positive experience.

Preparing for an active birth during pregnancy will lessen the likelihood of complications arising. It will also ensure that you approach the birth of your baby in optimal health, which will enhance and hasten your recovery, whatever happens. If you give birth actively you will want to move around freely during the early part, or first stage, of labor, choosing comfortable upright positions such as standing, walking, sitting, kneeling, or squatting. In between contractions you can find ways to rest in these positions, comfortably supported by pillows. As you approach the expulsive or second stage, during which your child can be born, you will continue to use the upright positions that are most comfortable or practical. At the end, for the actual birth, you can use a natural expulsive position (probably supported) like squatting or kneeling.

An active birth is instinctive. It involves your giving birth quite naturally and spontaneously through your own will and determination, having the complete freedom to use your body as you choose and to follow its urges. Active birth is an attitude of mind. It involves acceptance and trust in the natural function and involuntary nature of the birth process, as well as an attitude or appropriate positioning of your body. It is not merely a vaginal extraction in which the attendants are in control and you are a passive patient. It is more comfortable, safer, and more efficient than a passive "confinement." This is supported by the many scientific studies comparing women who are active in labor with those in a passive, recumbent position (see page 13).

Some women, left to themselves, will instinctively know what to do in labor, but most of us, having no example to follow, need to be made aware of the possibilities of using various upright positions in order to discover our instincts. This can easily be done by practicing during your pregnancy the birth positions and movements that are most appropriate and comfortable. The yoga-based exercises in this book will lead you towards your own instincts for labor and birth, while cultivating the right and natural body habits for a healthy pregnancy.

THE QUESTION OF BIRTH POSITIONS

A growing number of mothers, midwives, nurses, obstetricians, and childbirth educators are questioning certain modern labor and birth practices, and the passive role demanded of women in contemporary maternity care. One practice that is being criticized is the almost exclusive use of lying, or recumbent, positions for childbirth; these are known as supine, dorsal, and lithotomy positions. There is more than sufficient evidence that upright birth positions—kneeling, sitting, standing, and squatting—are more advantageous to both mother and child.

Position and movement in labor is an area of fundamental importance that has been, in the past, almost completely neglected by birth attendants in the management of labor, and therefore also by prenatal teachers in the preparation of women for birth. The customary choice of position determines the training of doctors and nurse-midwives. It determines their approach and the kind of environment in which women labor and give birth. It can also determine the outcome of the birth and the quality of the experience for both mother and baby.

MODERN WESTERN PRACTICE

Obstetric practice in the modern world usually defines birth as a medical, if not surgical, procedure. The normal practice in most hospitals has until recently been (and often still is) to place the laboring woman in bed on her back, at best propped up by pillows into a semireclining position, so that a monitor, drip, anesthetic, or all three can be conveniently applied. Later, just before the time of actual birth, she may be transferred to a delivery room and placed on an obstetric table, where her baby can be most conveniently "delivered" by her attendants, often with a forceps, vacuum extraction, episiotomy, or cesarean section.

Generally the choice of birth positions is predetermined by the hospital's approach to maternity care and its routine practices. Usually, the training of doctors takes the recumbent position for granted in specific obstetric practices, such as—

- The continuous assessment of fetal heart tones, uterine contractions, and other vital signs during labor through the use of electronic fetal monitors, which were designed for use in the recumbent position. Paradoxically, by requiring the supine position these often cause the fetal distress they are meant to detect.[1]
- Periodic vaginal examinations with the mother lying on her back. Where birth is active there is less need for vaginal examinations, as the progress of labor can usually be assessed by the mother's behavior. If

an internal examination is considered to be necessary, it can usually be done conveniently enough with the mother remaining upright.

- The use of sedatives, oxytocin, analgesics, and anesthesia during labor and delivery. If the mother is not lying down in the first place she is less likely to need pain-relieving drugs or oxytocin.
- The use of forceps or vacuum extraction, with episiotomy, for delivery, or the routine "controlling" of the delivery or "guarding" of the perineum. None of these practices are routinely needed in an active birth.

When such practices are routinely used, labor and birth are seen from the outset as a potentially pathological situation controlled by attendants and their technology rather than by the woman herself, her instincts, and her body.

No one will deny the enormous advantages of modern obstetrics when problems occur that may threaten the life of the mother or the baby, or both. The vast majority of labors, however, have the potential to be uncomplicated. Clearly, common sense in the management of normal labor has been completely obscured by the routine application of interventive obstetrics, resulting in a great increase in the number of forceps deliveries and cesarean sections.

In many countries in the developed world, most labors in hospitals are induced or followed by forceps delivery, (or both), and the cesarean rate is as high as 30 percent. In the United States, approximately 25 percent of births are cesarean, which reflects a 400 percent increase in 20 years.[2] In some hospitals, as many as one in three births are cesarean, and in some large teaching hospitals the figure is closer to 60 percent.

Among other practices, the rigid insistence on making women in labor lie on their backs contributes largely to these figures. It seems that a vicious circle arises: as soon as we begin to intervene in the natural process, the possibility of complication increases, and the need for intervention and for pain-relieving drugs becomes more prevalent. When a laboring woman is immobilized and required to lie on her back, the natural process is fundamentally disturbed, and the likelihood of problems occurring increases.

WHAT IS WRONG
WITH OBSTETRICALLY-MANAGED BIRTH?

Giving birth can, and usually does, involve hours of intense labor and a great deal of pain, effort, and endurance on your part. Naturally, the prospect is quite awesome, and you will probably approach the birth of your child with some fear and apprehension about what is to come.

To many women the prospect of a painless, effortless, managed birth might at first seem to be attractive. After all, you might ask, why suffer needlessly when medication and modern technology are readily available to make the birth easier, quicker, and less painful?

Regrettably, it is not as simple as all that. Every interventive obstetric technique has known side effects for mother and baby, while many subtle or long-term effects may not yet be apparent. When help is genuinely needed, the benefits of the intervention may well outweigh the risks. However, routine obstetric management tends to complicate birth unnecessarily.

We have known since the 1960s that all obstetric medications given to the mother, whether they are used to quell nausea, to induce labor, to relieve pain, or to anesthetize, do cross the placenta and do alter the baby's environment in the uterus, entering the baby's circulatory system and hence the baby's brain within seconds or minutes. Contrary to what many women are told, this includes regional anesthetics, commonly used in epidurals. These drugs will cross to the baby in small amounts and cause subtle but measurable neurobehavioral changes.[3]

The baby's central nervous system forms and develops rapidly in the last part of pregnancy, during the birth itself, and during infancy, and is susceptible to the effects of drugs given around the time of birth and after. We have only to recall the thalidomide tragedy to realize that the testing of the safety of these medications is often sorely inadequate. Of course, it is important also to bear in mind that babies vary in their vulnerability to the effects of these drugs and, in instances of real need, the judicious and minimal use of medication is usually successful. However, in prenatal clinics and hospitals, mothers are seldom informed about the hazards or side effects involved in taking such medications and are deluded into assuming that there are no risks involved.

Let us take a look at some examples of the most widely used medications for labor and birth, and their more common side effects. I have deliberately omitted the more severe and rare complications, but readers who are interested can look up the research reports.

The Promise of Pain Relief

Narcotics

The best-known of these drugs is Demerol. Used to "take the edge off" pain, these medications are usually given as intramuscular injections. Some women find they make labor more tolerable, and others that the drugs cause them to lose control. These drugs have possible side effects on the mother, such as nausea and dizziness, and they slow down the mother's breathing and respiration, hence reducing the baby's oxygen supply. To reduce the mother's nausea, they are often mixed with sedatives, and these too enter the baby's bloodstream and cause sleepiness.

It is now common knowledge that Demerol and similar drugs can depress the baby's respiratory system and jeopardize the start of breathing after birth.[4] Although medical personnel try to prevent breathing problems by timing the dosage of the drug to wear off sufficiently before birth, and by having other drugs available to reverse the narcotic's effects, the baby must sometimes be resuscitated.

Traces of these medications sometimes remain in the baby's circulatory system after birth, so that, in addition to adjusting to life outside the womb, the baby's system has the added burden of detoxification.[5] Because these traces remain in the baby's body for several weeks, they can also depress the baby's sucking reflex and can affect the initiation of breastfeeding and mother-infant bonding.[6]

Epidural Anesthesia

This is the common name for the injection of a regional anesthetic into the epidural space between two lumbar vertebrae in the lower spine. When the injection works, the result is a blocking of pain impulses, bringing numbness from the waist to the thighs or down to the toes.

While the drugs used for epidurals do not affect the baby as Demerol does, we know that they enter the baby's circulation and brain tissues within minutes.[7] Their immediate and long-term effects on the baby's neurological development are relatively unknown and direly under-re-searched, despite the widespread use of this form of pain relief worldwide.

Side effects for the mother, such as severe headaches following the birth, can occasionally occur (these are caused by accidental penetration of the membrane surrounding the spinal cord by the injection needle), and a lowering of maternal blood pressure is common.

An epidural certainly increases the need for obstetric intervention. If the mother is immobile and reclining, her contractions tend to be less efficient. Labor is often much longer and may need to be artificially stimulated with an oxytocic drip.

All these factors contribute to a lessening of the blood supply to and from the uterus, so fetal distress (lack of oxygen) is far more likely. Sometimes the pelvic muscles become limp and do not help the baby to rotate in the usual way (with the added disadvantage of the baby's not having the help of gravity).

An epidural can also inhibit the mother's ability to push her baby out spontaneously, and, in one way or another, increase the risk of a forceps delivery, a vacuum extraction, or a cesarean section.

At the Garden Hospital in North London, where mothers give birth actively with the help of a midwife, the forceps rate rarely rises above 5 percent and drugs are used only in cases of unavoidable distress or to save a life. In contrast, in U.S. hospitals where epidurals are the norm, the incidence of forceps delivery can be as high as 65 percent, according to Doris Haire.[8] A forceps delivery can be traumatic for both mother and child and can occasionally result in injury to the baby.[9]

Although at times the total freedom from pain offered by an epidural may be indispensable, it is important to weigh this advantage against the attendant risks, which are considerable. Occasionally the price of a few hours of comfort is a damaged baby; often it is a complicated birth.[10]

So, might it not be better in the long run to learn how to use your body to release, minimize, and transform the pain of labor, and to have access to a pool of warm water or a shower—effective and totally harmless ways to reduce pain? If an epidural is really needed, then the dose should be as low as possible to reduce the attendant risks.

Stimulating Labor

Pitocin

This drug may be used to initiate labor or to strengthen contractions once labor has begun. A powerful synthetic hormone, Pitocin is introduced into a vein in the mother's arm via an intravenous drip.

Normally, when the uterus contracts, the blood vessels that carry blood to the placenta are temporarily constricted. In between contractions, blood is stored in the placenta to keep up a constant supply to the baby during contractions. When contractions are stimulated by Pitocin they tend to be longer, stronger, and closer together than in a normal labor. The periods of constriction are therefore longer than usual, so that the overall oxygen supply to the baby is reduced and fetal distress is therefore more likely. Doris Haire compares the situation to "holding an infant under water and allowing the infant to come to the surface to gasp for air but not to breathe."[11]

The incidence of postnatal jaundice in babies whose mothers' labors are induced is also thought to be higher.[12]

In addition, strong contractions usually occur as soon as the drip begins to work, so the gradual buildup in intensity of a normal labor is absent. This often means that the mother cannot cope with the pain of the stronger contractions and needs pain relief, so the baby ends up with the combined effect of painkillers and the drugs used for induction.

Of course, continuous fetal monitoring is usually necessary with all these risks, so the snowball effect continues as one intervention necessitates another.

Studies have shown that there is no advantage in routinely inducing births that are "overdue." A failed induction frequently ends up as a cesarean section.[13]

Would it not be better to reserve this option as a last resort, and to discover how to change position to stimulate contractions, or how to improve the birthing environment so the mother can secrete her own natural hormones? Allowing the normal physiology to unfold without disturbance is the most effective way to ensure that the mother will secrete her own hormones.

BIRTH BEFORE OBSTETRICS

Historical studies show the prevalent use of vertical positions—kneeling, squatting, standing, or sitting postures—with many variations and as many methods of support.

There is evidence going back thousands of years of the bodily positions taken in childbirth. The head of a silver pin from Luristan in Persia, first millennium B.C., depicts a squatting mother. The remains of a clay statue of 5750 B.C. from a shrine at Çatal Huyuk, a Copper Age (Chalcolithic) city in present-day Turkey, shows a goddess giving birth in the same position, as does an 8½-inch Aztec stone fertility figure from Mexico. A relic of the Mound Builders of present-day eastern Arkansas, a pre-Columbian culture of unknown date, shows a woman squatting with her hands on her thighs. The Egyptian hieroglyph meaning "to give birth" shows a mother squatting. A relief from the temple of Kom Ombo, a town on the Nile in Upper Egypt, shows a woman giving birth in the kneeling position. Birth in the same position can be seen in a marble figure from Sparta, dated about 500 B.C. In ancient China and Japan, women customarily gave birth in the kneeling position on a straw mat. Although most ancient representations of birth show the posture used as the baby emerges, positions used during labor can also be traced.

In the Old Testament, Exod. 1:16 contains these words: "When ye do the office of a midwife to the Hebrew women, and see them upon the stools. . . ." A Corinthian vase depicts a woman in labor seated on a chair with a horseshoe-shaped seat. An early Greek relief and a Roman marble bas-relief both show a woman giving birth on a stool supported by two assistants. The birthstool was recommended for uncomplicated labors by Soranus in the early part of the second century A.D., as well as many subsequent writers. He described it as being "in a form like a barber's chair but with a crescent-shaped opening in the seat through which the child may fall." The first birthstools may have been rocks or logs, which developed over time into complex, adjustable chairs with many varied devices.

With or without a birthstool or birthchair, women giving birth in ancient representations use upright postures and are usually supported by one or more attendants while the midwife receives the baby.

FROM BIRTHCHAIR TO BED TO DELIVERY TABLE

In the Western world, the birthstool or birthchair remained indispensably part of the equipment of most midwives up to the middle of the eighteenth century. Each wealthy household had its own stool, while among the poor a stool was transported from house to house. The birthstools of royalty were carved and ornamented with jewels. Sixteenth-century Dutch, German, and French drawings show the great use of birthstools, as do Chinese drawings of the same period. Even today, a birthchair is still used by some Egyptian women.

The first known advocate for the recumbent position in childbirth was Aristotle. In *The Experienced Midwife* (350 B.C.), he wrote: "The bed ought to be ordered that the woman, being ready to be delivered, should lie on her back upon it, having her body in a convenient posture; that is, her head and breast a little raised so that she be between lying and sitting."[14] Other classical authors, however, recommended upright postures.

In the early-seventeenth century in France, two brothers named Chamberlen invented the forceps. The best way to perform a forceps delivery is to have the woman lying down. This invention was jealously guarded by the Chamberlens, who performed their deliveries shrouded by black drapes, but the obstetric fashion for aristocratic women to give birth in recumbent positions became firmly entrenched, especially after Madame de Montespan, mistress of Louis XIV, lay down to give birth so her lover could watch the event from behind a curtain. In the same century, François Mauriceau became the leading figure in French obstetrics. He scorned the use of the birthchair and, following Aristotle, advocated childbirth in bed, lying on the back. As the physician took over from the midwife in the birth chamber and forceps gained popularity, the birthchair lost favor. By the end of the eighteenth century, little more was heard of it.

In the nineteenth century, Queen Victoria was the first woman in England to have chloroform while giving birth. Delivery under anesthetic further established the lying-down position, on the back or on the side. Birth positions that suited the convenience of the attendants who performed these procedures became the only choice, and the practice of confining a woman to bed for the major part of her labor, and then to an obstetric table for delivery, eventually spread throughout the West.

The birthchair had given way to the bed and the delivery tables of the nineteenth and twentieth centuries. Women were flat on their backs, a position that made them passive and controllable, and although this offered a fine view to the attendant, it was in total defiance of the force of gravity and the joyous independence that comes from naturally and instinctively giving birth actively, on one's own two feet.

ETHNOLOGICAL EVIDENCE

Women in traditional societies have adopted various birth positions through the customs of their peoples and, more important, through their instinct. Some forty positions have been recorded, and their relative merits have been much disputed. Women of different societies squat, kneel, stand, lean, sit, or lie on the belly; so too do they vary their positions among the stages of labor and in difficult labors.

In his book *Labour Among Primitive Peoples*, written in 1883, Dr G. J. Englemann was one of the first to investigate the various positions assumed in labor and childbirth by the world's peoples.[15] He found that the four principal positions were squatting, kneeling (including the all-fours and knee-chest positions), standing, and semirecumbent. Ethnologists entirely confirm the evidence of the historians. Whatever the society under observation—African, American, Asian, or other—upright positions always predominate, with a great variety of means of support. Figures reveal that, for the most part, women throughout most of the world today still labor and deliver in some form of upright or crouching position, usually supported. Their numbers are declining rapidly, however, with the loss of traditional practices and the introduction of modern hospitals throughout the developing countries.

RECENT STUDIES

Over the past few decades, as disillusionment with the routine application of high-tech obstetrics has increased, researchers all over the world have begun to explore normal physiological birth. Documented evidence has been available for over fifty years on the physiological advantages of labor in upright or crouching positions. Certain principles of physics apply to childbirth, and these are opposed when a woman gives birth lying down. The benefits of squatting were radiographically confirmed in the 1930s, when it was shown that the cross-sectional surface area of the birth canal may increase by as much as 30 percent when a woman changes from lying down on her back to the squatting position.[16] And it is nearly thirty years since Scott and Kerr demonstrated the disadvantages of having the weight of a full-term pregnant uterus pressing down on the back. When the woman lies supine, the weight of the contracting uterus reduces the placental blood flow by compressing the large artery of the heart (the descending aorta) and the large veins leading to the heart (inferior vena cava). This is a clinical fact that should not be ignored by anyone involved with childbirth.[17]

Most recent studies have revealed definite advantages to a woman when she is walking about and keeping upright during labor. The few researchers, and they are a very small minority, who have found no measurable advantage, all conclude that there is at least no *dis*advantage to being active and using upright positions during labor.

The majority of studies have established a control group and an experimental group. They have usually required that the control group remain supine or in some recumbent position in bed, and that the experimental group assume an upright posture—sitting, squatting, kneeling, or walking about. But other studies, which seem more convincing, have used the women as their own controls, asking them to alternate every thirty minutes between two positions—horizontal and upright—during the first and second stages of labor. These alternative approaches to examining the effect of position during labor both reveal positive results in favor of active upright labor and deliveries.

During the 1970s many such studies were carried out in various parts of the world. In 1977, a study at the Birmingham (England) Maternity Hospital compared a group of women who walked about during labor with a group that lay down throughout most of labor. The results showed that the duration of labor was significantly shorter, the need for analgesics far less, and the incidence of fetal heart abnormalities markedly smaller in the ambulant group than in the recumbent group. Women walking about also reported less pain with uterine contractions, and they felt more comfortable upright. The researchers concluded convincingly that walking about during labor, especially early labor, should be encouraged.[18]

Other studies, in the United States, Latin America, and elsewhere, confirmed that when laboring women were upright and moving about the following advantages ensued:

- Uterine contractions were more intense (that is, stronger).
- Uterine contractions were more regular and frequent.
- The cervix (the neck of the uterus) dilated, or opened, more efficiently.
- The women relaxed more completely between contractions.
- The pressure of the baby's head on the cervix during the resting phase between uterine contractions was consistently higher.
- The first and second stages of labor were shorter (some studies showed they were over 40 percent shorter in the upright group).
- The women felt greater comfort and less stress and pain, and so required less analgesics.
- The incidence of fetal distress in labor was lower, and the condition of the newborn was generally better.
- Women felt they were contributing something to their labor and felt relieved from the boredom and degradation of lying down connected to equipment.[19]

Even though these studies were carried out in birthing environments that could have been improved, with women who had no special preparation, the results were impressive when only the women's posture was changed.

WHY IS ACTIVE BIRTH BETTER?

What explains the fact that women have easier labors and births when they move about and assume upright positions? Common sense and recent studies suggest that these are the advantages to the upright mother and her baby:

1. The pull of gravity—that is, the Earth's downward gravitational force—assists uterine contractions and bearing-down efforts. Since it is easier for any object to fall towards the Earth's surface than to slide parallel to it (according to Newton's Law of Gravity), it is mechanically more advantageous to expel an unborn baby towards the Earth than to expel it along the horizon. In an upright position, such as standing, squatting, or kneeling, the mother's body is in harmony with the downward force of gravity. When she lies down, her involuntary efforts to expel the baby

are inhibited; she must strain harder to push the baby "uphill," and she is more likely to need the help of forceps. Dr. Peter Dunn, of Southmead Hospital in Bristol, England, writes of the recumbent position for labor: "No animal species adopts such a disadvantageous posture during such an important and critical event."[20]

2. The drive angle of the uterus—that is, the angle between the long axis of the unborn baby's spinal column and that of the mother's spinal column—is greater when the mother is upright, so less effort is demanded from the uterus. The uterus tends to tilt forward when it contracts. In an upright position the mother can lean forward, thereby assisting her uterus to work without resistance, but if she is lying down or leaning back, the uterus has to work harder, since it is pulled back by gravity when it tries to tilt forward during a contraction (see page 117). A muscle working against gravity tends to tire and ache more easily, so leaning forward is an efficient way to reduce pain and the need for analgesics.

3. The entrance of the baby's head to the inlet of the mother's pelvis is easiest when she is upright, because in this position the pelvic inlet points forward and the outlet faces downwards. This provides the baby the best angle of descent, in relation to gravity, through the pelvic canal.

4. The direct application of the baby's head to the dilating cervix is also assisted when the mother is upright. With each contraction the unborn baby tends to sink downwards towards the cervix. Between contractions, as the mother rests in an upright position, the pressure on the cervix is sustained by the weight of the baby's body and the mother's abdominal contents. This results in more efficient and faster dilation.

5. Placental circulation is improved, giving a better oxygen supply to the fetus. Lying on one's back is the one position that causes compression of the major abdominal blood vessels along the spinal column. Compression of the large artery of the heart (descending aorta) can cause fetal distress by hindering blood circulation around the uterus and the placenta. Compression of the large veins leading to the heart (inferior vena cava) blocks the returning blood flow, contributing to hypotension and the possibility of maternal hemorrhage.

6. The pelvic nerves that supply the pelvic cavity and uterus arise from the lower part of the spinal cord and enter the pelvis through the sacrum. When a woman avoids lying on her back, there is no direct pressure on these nerves, so she feels less pain. When she puts her weight on her sacrum, the nerves are compressed and her pain is increased.

7. During pregnancy hormones soften the ligaments around the pelvic

joints to make the joints more flexible. As long as the mother is upright for the birth, the pelvic joints are free to expand, move, and adjust to the shape of the baby's descending head. When the mother squats, the sacrum is free to move, allowing the anterior-interior diameter of the pelvic outlet to widen by as much as 30 percent more than it would if the mother's weight were resting directly on it—that is, if she were semireclining. The sacrococcygeal joint, the joint between the sacrum and the coccyx or tailbone, also softens in pregnancy; it is designed to swivel backwards to widen the outlet of the pelvis as the baby emerges. Of course, this is impossible if the mother is sitting on her coccyx.

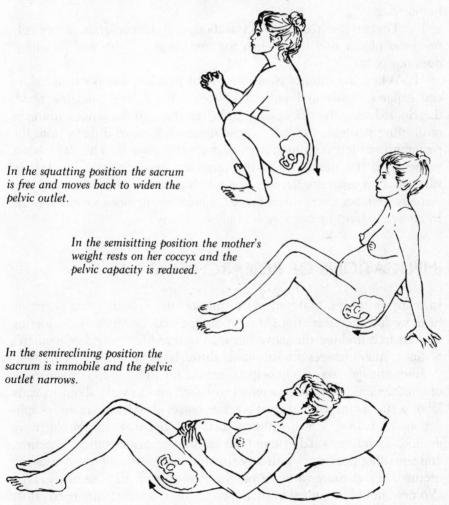

In the squatting position the sacrum is free and moves back to widen the pelvic outlet.

In the semisitting position the mother's weight rests on her coccyx and the pelvic capacity is reduced.

In the semireclining position the sacrum is immobile and the pelvic outlet narrows.

8. When the mother is upright during the second stage, there is less direct pressure on the baby's neck vertebrae as the head passes under the pubic arch and the neck extends backwards (see diagram on page 29). Although no studies have yet been done, experienced parents and birth attendants will observe that actively born babies have better head control immediately after birth. This facilitates the "rooting reflex" for breastfeeding and also enhances motor development after birth.

9. Upright positions facilitate the successful and spontaneous separation of the placenta and reduce both the need to assist the delivery of the placenta by pulling on the cord and the risk of postpartum infection or hemorrhage.[21]

10. There is less likelihood of infection, as fluids can drain more easily from the uterus after birth when the mother is upright, and "pooling" does not occur.

11. When the mother is in an upright position, the perineal tissues can expand evenly and pull back around the baby's emerging head, thereby reducing the risk of tearing. When she is in the semireclining or semisitting position, the baby's head descends forward directly onto the perineum, which is immobilized and cannot expand. The situation is worsened if the mother is in the lithotomy position with her legs in stirrups. This separates the legs to a much greater extent than usual and actually stretches the perineal tissues, increasing the need for episiotomy. In an active birth episiotomy is rarely necessary.

IMPLICATIONS OF RESEARCH FINDINGS

In many countries, maternity care and prenatal education are changing to allow and encourage upright positions for labor and birth. Considering the research findings on active birth, as well as the strength of women's instinct, such changes are inevitable throughout the United States.[22]

Since changes in position help to increase the strength and effectiveness of contractions, to allow a woman to be up and to walk about in early labor seems a rational and good practice especially if there are no complications. A woman's own instincts dictate to her that she should move around. Standing, walking about, and assuming various sitting, kneeling, and squatting positions, with any suitable means of support, causes the uterus to exert more pressure on the fetus and in turn on the cervix. Women should be guided by their own feelings, comfort, and need rather than by hospital convenience and obstetric fashion. Freedom of one's body is necessary to find those positions that traditionally have been used to facilitate labor and delivery—positions that will assist one to attain maximum comfort, relaxation, ease, and control.

There is an infinite range of possible positions and no best order among them. The laboring woman's instincts tell her to keep searching for the most effective, efficient, and comfortable positions. The common need among women instinctively to keep changing positions will one day have to be universally recognized. This involves a different attitude to the management of labor, to maternity care generally, and to prenatal preparation.

A prospective mother needs not only knowledge of pregnancy, labor, and delivery and the growth and development of babies, but also adequate physical preparation: she needs to become familiar and comfortable with various upright positions and to learn what their effects are in labor so that she will be able to help herself at the birth. The emphasis during pregnancy needs to be on developing trust and confidence in her own body and on learning to discover her instincts for childbirth and mothering. Her emotional and physical readiness for birth and her self-empowerment in pregnancy will become as important as good prenatal medical care.

An Ideal Position for Birth?

Being free to change position during labor is more important than finding a single best position. It is unlikely that any woman would elect to remain in one position throughout labor. However, squatting is most closely allied with nature's laws; it is therefore known as "the physiological position." A position is physiologically effective when (1) there is no compression on the vena cava or the aorta, and (2) the pelvis is fully mobilized.

Supported squatting seems to be especially efficient at the end of the second stage, when the baby is being born. The squatting position produces—

- maximum pressure inside the pelvis,
- minimal muscular effort,
- optimal relaxation of the perineum,
- optimal oxygen supply to the fetus, and
- the most efficient angle of descent in relation to gravity.

A supported standing squat is the most practical position for a vaginal breech delivery. By maximizing the help of gravity, it reduces delay between delivery of the umbilicus and the head.

Also useful is the all-fours position. The presenting part rotates inside the pelvis more easily when a woman is on all fours. This position can be especially useful if the baby is lying posterior or the birth is very fast.

None of the women in the recent studies were prenatally prepared to gain ease and comfort in the squatting, kneeling, crouching, or all-fours position. How much better the upright women might have fared if they had the additional benefit of physical preparation! But a controlled study of women prepared for active birth has yet to be done.

IDEAL MATERNITY CARE?

At the maternity unit in the general hospital in Pithiviers, France, Michel Odent and his staff founded a setting for women to be active in labor. Here, beginning in 1960, laboring women had the freedom to follow their instincts in walking about and finding comfortable positions. Dr. Odent, the midwives, and expectant mothers discovered many means of gravity-effective support that proved, over the years, to be tremendously helpful in easing labor and expecially delivery.

The aim at Pithiviers was to "demedicalize" pregnancy and birth. Prenatal visits were limited to the minimum of four required by French law. However, mothers and their families were encouraged to attend regular informal singing groups so that the hospital and midwives would be familiar to them long before the birth. Prenatal yoga classes were also available at the hospital.

Odent's concept of obstetrics—that the normal physiology should not be disturbed—was very different from conventional practice, aimed at control. Also, the physical and the social environment was unusual: the birthing room had a homelike rather than a hospital atmosphere. It was simply furnished, in earth tones, without furniture suggestive of any particular position.

In this unit about one thousand deliveries a year took place. Professional care was the responsibility of Odent and six midwives. The midwives worked in pairs; a pair was on duty for 48 continuous hours, followed by four days off. Each client was given a room to call her own throughout her stay, and there were few rules. As labor advanced, she walked to the birthing room, which had a low platform with many cushions, and a wooden squatting stool. In the birthing room she was encouraged to remain active and change her position as many times as she wished. She could walk about, sit on the birthstool, get on all fours, squat, and lean on her husband or the midwife for physical support. If she liked, she could take a warm bath or relax in a small pool that was available, for water was regarded as an important aid in labor.

In labor, drugs such as Pitocin and Demerol, and obstetric interventions such as cesareans, episiotomies, and vacuum extractions, were used only in rare circumstances. Membranes were not artificially ruptured. Electronic fetal heart monitoring was not used at all, and vaginal examinations were kept to a minimum.

Most women adopted an upright position for delivery, usually a supported squat. Some gave birth on the birthstool or on the low platform, and some gave birth in water. With the appropriate supported squat and the minimal disturbance of the expulsive reflex, there were no unnecessary perineal tears, and episiotomies were rare.

After the birth, the baby's bath, and the delivery of the placenta, the mother walked with her husband and her newborn back to her own room.

Women were not screened for admission to the maternity unit at Pithiviers. In fact, some came specifically because they were "high-risk"—they had had, for example, previous cesarean or breech deliveries—and were for this reason unable to arrange vaginal births elsewhere. Yet Pithiviers's perinatal mortality rate was below the French average for

Data from 1815 Births at Pithiviers, 1982–83

	N	Percentage
Women with previous cesareans	66	3.6
Vaginal births after cesareans	36	2.0
Cesareans	125	6.9
Perinatal deaths[a]	14	0.8
Vacuum extractions[b]	89	4.9
Episiotomies	106	5.8
Manual removal of placenta	16	0.9
Transfer to pediatrics	27	1.5

Source: Michel Odent, "Towards Less Mechanized Childbirth: The Pithiviers Experience," in *Advances in International Maternal and Child Health* 5, ed. D. B. Jelliffe and E. F. P. Jelliffe (Oxford: Clarendon Press, 1985).

[a]All deaths after 6 months of intrauterine life and before 7 days after birth.

[b]Forceps were never used.

each year from 1962 to 1982, and, despite the unit's limited use of interventions, there were no maternal deaths.[23] The general statistics from Pithiviers compare very favorably with those of conventional hospitals, in 1983 and today.

The maternity unit at Pithiviers was so successful, Odent says, because the staff's aim was to try, at least, not to disturb the natural physiological processes of birth, and, at best, to facilitate them. Here was a maternity-care setting close to ideal. It had the safety of hospital delivery as well as a comfortable, homelike birthing room and a relaxed atmosphere. It was free of the frustrating regulations and limitations of most hospitals, for the staff observed and understood the instinctive behavior of women in labor. The attendants were well known to the mother and were constantly available during labor and delivery. Fathers who wished to share the experience helped to support their partners. Women had the freedom to move and adopt any position they found comfortable, and drugs and interventions during labor were rarely needed.

Odent now works in London with mothers giving birth at home—the only place, he now maintains, where a woman has the degree of privacy needed to allow maximal efficiency of the physiological and hormonal responses.[24] As a result of his example of Pithiviers, however, many maternity units have been established along similar lines throughout the world, and these units continue to show strikingly good results compared with hospitals where obstetric management is routine.

One of these pioneering maternity units is North London's Garden Hospital, with which I have a close working association.[25] For more than 10 years, this small unit has exemplified active birth in a homelike hospital environment. Pregnant women prepare for birth using the methods suggested in this book, and they attend yoga classes with my colleague Lolly Stirk and me as well as weekly social meetings with the midwives and obstetricians. They also visit the labor ward each time they attend the prenatal clinic. In labor, women have the freedom to behave instinctively and the support of an excellent team of familiar midwives. Pain-relieving medications are freely available to those who prefer to use them, but most mothers give birth actively and naturally. A deep water pool is available for use during labor and birth.

A recent accounting of births at the Garden Hospital shows a very low rate of obstetrical interventions (see table).

If the majority of women at Pithiviers and the Garden Hospital can safely experience natural, active birth, why can't women everywhere?

Data from 316 Births at the Garden Hospital, 1990

	N	Percentage
Primiparas (first-time mothers)	142	44.9
Active births[a]	228	72.2
Water births	67	21.2
Previous cesareans[b]	18	5.7
Vaginal births after cesareans	9	2.8
Breech births[c]	11	3.5
Perinatal death	1	0.3
Women using water pool in labor	194	61.4
Induced labors (using Pitocin)[d]	11	3.5
Augmented labors (using Pitocin)	23	7.3
Demerol for pain relief	1	0.3
Epidural anesthesia[e]	55	17.4
General anesthesia	14	4.4
Cesareans	43	13.6
Forceps deliveries[f]	20	6.3
Episiotomies	22	7.0
Manual removal of placenta	1	0.3

[a]These mothers moved about and used upright positions, and had no drugs or other obstetrical interventions. The figures include water births.

[b]Of these women 9 gave birth vaginally, 9 by cesarean (some of these cesareans were elective).

[c]Seven were vaginal births, without forceps or other intervention; 4 were cesarean births. Two breech babies were twins, and both were born actively.

[d]One labor was induced after the fetus had been determined dead.

[e]Most women who had epidurals labored actively until receiving anesthesia, then were helped to give birth in upright squatting positions.

[f]Vacuum extraction was never used.

YOUR RESPONSIBILITY

If having the freedom to move and adopt upright positions makes sense to you, and you want to give birth actively but do not have access to a maternity unit like the Garden Hospital or Pithiviers, what can you do? You will have to make the possibility of an active birth your own responsibility; you will have to prepare your body to find ease and comfort in upright positions, and, whether you wish to give birth at home or in the hospital, you will have to find a midwife or doctor who will support you in giving birth actively without the conventional interventions.

In parts of Britain, Europe, North and South America, Australia, New Zealand, and elsewhere, increasing numbers of mothers, doctors, midwives, and prenatal teachers are putting active birth into practice and teaching others to do the same. Small groups are springing up everywhere, spreading their message by word of mouth. (You can write the Active Birth Centre for a list of such groups in the United States; see "Resources.") The women who form these groups have experienced active birth without drugs, without episiotomies, and without tears. Women who join them prepare themselves to give birth actively by finding prenatal teachers who encourage them and doctors and midwives, maternity units, and staff who are prepared to assist them to move about and use upright positions.

One of these alternative birth groups may be able to help you find a supportive attendant. In some areas, however, it may be impossible to find a birth attendant experienced with active birth. In this case you will need to be a pioneer; you'll need to introduce your birth attendant to the idea of active birth. By agreeing to accept help if a problem arises or if you feel you need it during labor, you may be able to persuade your attendant to let you take responsibility when you get to the hospital. Then prepare yourself very well—by following the suggestions in this book, reading other books, taking the best childbirth class you can find, and doing everything else you can to empower yourself during pregnancy. The support of your mate may be very helpful, or you can select a friend or relative as birth partner. By practicing various active birthing positions together, you can approach the birth as a team, with confidence and know-how.

In this way many mothers in the United Kingdom have impressed their birth attendants and thus inspired change within the maternity system, while enjoying their experience and retaining the security of obstetric backup. The balance of power can gradually shift this way, until real freedom of choice becomes available to all women. Although it is not easy to have a baby at a time when obstetric practices are changing so much, the challenge of taking responsibility for your own baby's birth can be exciting, and you may find that your birth attendant is willing to observe and learn from your example.

It is wise to discuss the ideas in this book with your doctor or midwife early in pregnancy, if possible. As you read this book it will be helpful to list important issues so that you and your birth attendant can go through them together, and then bring a copy of your list to the hospital for easy reference by the nurse, doctor, or midwife during labor. When labor starts it may help to request a nurse who is enthusiastic about natural birth and who has had previous experience in the use of upright postures.

2 | Your Body in Pregnancy

THE PELVIC ORGANS

Your uterus lies deep inside your abdominal cavity, between the bladder in front and the rectum behind. These three are known as the pelvic organs. Your abdominal cavity extends from your diaphragm, beneath your lungs, to the muscles of the floor of your pelvis.

Before pregnancy your uterus is a small, hollow muscular organ, shaped like an inverted pear, measuring roughly 3 inches by 2 inches by 1 inch. Extending to each side from the top part, or *fundus*, are two narrow canals, the *fallopian tubes*, and these end in finger-like projections called *fimbria*, which surround your ovaries on either side and draw up the ripe ovum after you ovulate. The lower part, or mouth, of the uterus is called the *cervix*. About 1½ inches long, the cervix projects into the vagina and opens up during labor to allow your child to be born. During pregnancy your cervix is closed, and the narrow opening is sealed with a mucous plug.

The uterus is the principal organ involved in pregnancy and childbirth. Your child is conceived in one of its fallopian tubes, implanted within

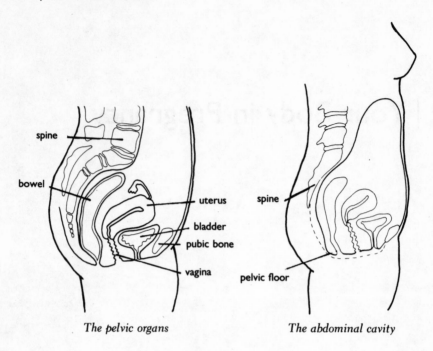

The pelvic organs   *The abdominal cavity*

its cavity, and, at the appropriate time, expelled by it through your vagina into the outside world.

The average length of pregnancy is considered to be 40 weeks from the first day of your last period. During this time your uterus increases in size to about 12 inches by 9 inches by 9 inches. Its weight increases from 3½ ounces to over 2 pounds at full term, and the amount of fluid it contains grows from a quarter of a teaspoon to approximately 1½ pints.

During the first 16 weeks of pregnancy, the expansion of your uterus is caused almost entirely by the growth of its tissues owing to hormonal stimulation. The uterus becomes a thick-walled organ, circular in shape and protected and cradled by the bones of your pelvis. Around 16 weeks you will begin to feel the "quickening" movements of your child within the womb.

About the twentieth week the organ's tissue growth almost ceases, and the uterus thenceforth expands because the muscle fibers are stretched by the growing child. At the very end of pregnancy the lower segment of the uterus stretches most, which is why a low-lying placenta will tend to rise

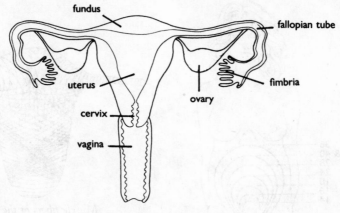

The maternal organs

as the uterine walls lengthen at the base. The walls of the uterus become thinner, and in the latter half of the pregnancy you can feel your child's body quite easily from outside. Your uterus becomes more oval in shape and moves up into your abdomen as your child grows.

As the uterus enlarges, its position changes. At 12 weeks the fundus, or top of the uterus, is just above your pelvic inlet. At 16 weeks, the fundus is nearly halfway to your navel, which it reaches at the eighteenth week. At 36 weeks, the top part of your uterus is lying just below your diaphragm, at the level of the lower end of your breastbone. During the last few weeks it drops a little lower as your baby settles into position for birth.

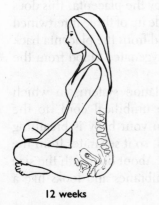
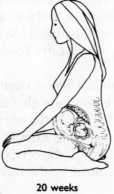
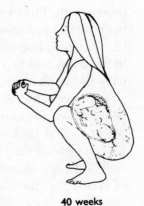

12 weeks   20 weeks   40 weeks

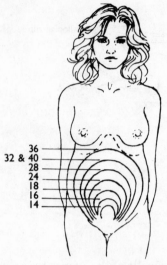

32 & 40
36
28
24
18
16
14

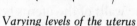
Varying levels of the uterus

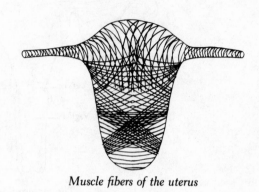
Muscle fibers of the uterus

Your uterus is a sack-shaped muscle consisting of a network of muscle fibers running in all directions, longitudinal, oblique, and circular.

During pregnancy your baby, lying within the uterus, is connected from the navel by the umbilical cord to the placenta, which is attached to the wall of your uterus. The placenta draws nourishment for your child from your bloodstream and, simultaneously, passes waste products back to you. The placenta usually implants in the upper segment of the uterus towards the back; sometimes it implants in front or lower down on the uterine wall. Provided the cervix is not covered by the placenta, this does not present a problem. The umbilical cord is made up of three intertwined blood vessels, one vein carrying oxygenated blood from the placenta back to the baby, and two arteries, which carry de-oxygenated blood from the baby to the placenta.

Your baby has an independent blood circulation system, in which blood flows all around the body, through the umbilical cord, to the placenta, and back again. After the birth, when your baby is breathing independently, the placenta is no longer needed, so it separates from the wall of the uterus and passes through the cervix. About one-sixth the size of your baby, the placenta is lined by the membranes and looks like a large piece of liver. If it is spread out and examined, one can see that it is a network of blood vessels, rather like the roots of a tree.

A membranous bag surrounds your baby, the placenta, and the cord. It also contains approximately 1½ pints of amniotic fluid—the waters within which your baby lies. These waters protect your baby from shock or infection and are constantly being replenished by your body.

At full term (at the end of pregnancy), the main function of your uterus is to empty itself. During labor the uterus contracts at regular intervals and gradually opens up at its base (the cervix) to allow your baby to pass through. Once it has opened, it contracts powerfully to expel your baby and the placenta, the membranes, and all contents of the uterus. (The placenta and membranes are called the "afterbirth.") In the hours and weeks after the birth, your uterus continues to contract rhythmically, stimulated by hormones. Your baby sucking on the breast will stimulate the release of these hormones. The uterus gradually shrinks back to its original shape and size and will expel all the blood-rich lining, which was used to nourish your baby. By the end of the sixth week after birth, your uterus will have completed its task and will be back to normal.

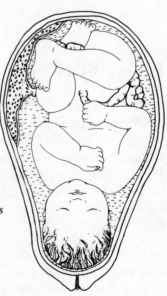

A baby at term, surrounded by waters and membranes with cord and placenta

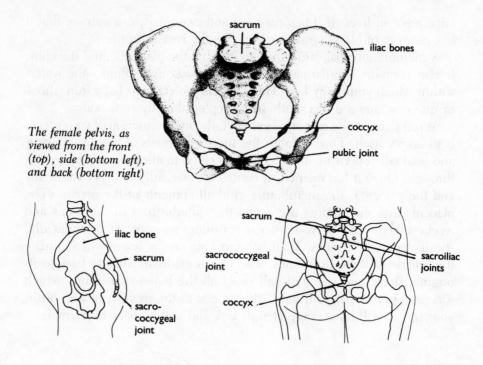

The female pelvis, as viewed from the front (top), side (bottom left), and back (bottom right)

sacrum

iliac bones

coccyx

pubic joint

sacrum

iliac bone

sacrum

sacrococcygeal joint

coccyx

sacroiliac joints

sacro-coccygeal joint

THE PELVIC BONES

Your pelvis is the part of your body most directly involved with giving birth. It is the bony passage through which your baby passes as it is born. During pregnancy your body produces hormones that soften the joints to increase their flexibility and thereby assist the birth of your child. By regularly practicing the exercises recommended in the next chapter, you can make the most of this natural flexibility and be at your physical best for giving birth.

Try this:

1. Kneel on the floor and explore your pelvis from the outside. Place your hands on your hips (*a*) and find the iliac crests—two bony points at your sides—and follow their curved rim with your thumbs around to the back. Feel your pubic bone in front, your sacrum (the back wall of the pelvis) and coccyx (tailbone) at the back.

2. Sit on your hands and feel your two buttock bones (*b*).

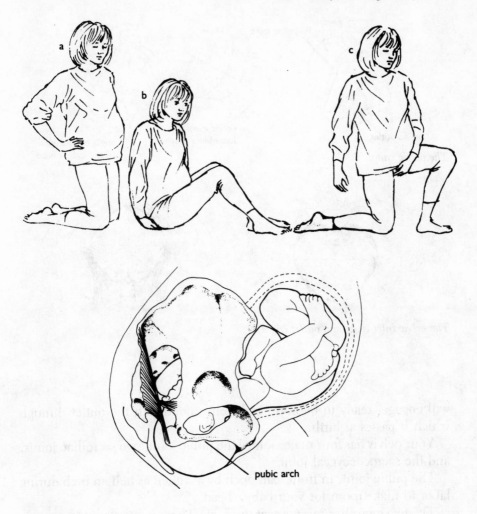

pubic arch

3. Kneel, then lift up one foot so that you are half-kneeling and half-squatting. Explore your pubic arch. Feel its curve extending from your buttock bones under your pubic bone. Your baby's head will pass under this arch as it is born (c).

Your pelvis is shaped internally like a curved funnel—exactly the right shape to accommodate your baby's head as it passes through during labor. When you examine the structure of a female pelvis apart from the rest of the body, from above you see the pelvic inlet in which your baby's head

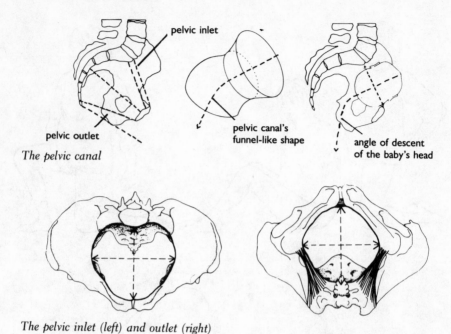

The pelvic canal

pelvic inlet

pelvic outlet

pelvic canal's funnel-like shape

angle of descent of the baby's head

The pelvic inlet (left) and outlet (right)

will engage, ready to be born; and from underneath the outlet through which it passes at birth.

Your pelvis has four major joints: the pubic joint, two sacroiliac joints, and the sacrococcygeal joint.

The pubic joint, in front, can open by as much as half an inch during labor to make room for your baby's head.

The two sacroiliac joints are at the back. These joints expand from side to side and also move in a pivot-like way to increase the area of the pelvic canal and adapt to the shape of the descending head of your baby as it passes through the pelvis.

The sacrococcygeal joint is between your coccyx and your sacrum. This joint loosens during pregnancy so that your coccyx can move out of the way as your baby is born. When you bend forward, as in squatting or the all-fours position, your sacrum and coccyx lift up, opening and expanding the pelvic outlet. When you bend backwards or recline, you narrow the pelvic outlet by as much as 30 percent. This is one of the reasons reclining is the worst position for giving birth.

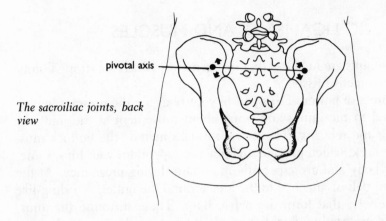

The sacroiliac joints, back view

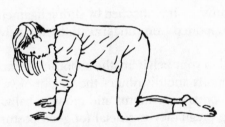

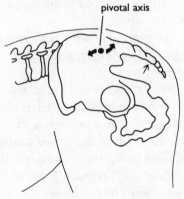

When you bend forward, the sacrum lifts up and the pelvic outlet widens.

When you lean back, the sacrum tucks in and the pelvic outlet narrows.

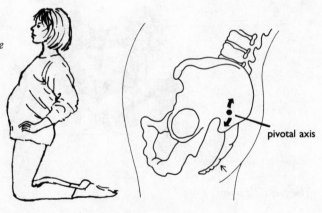

THE PELVIC LIGAMENTS AND MUSCLES

The pelvic joints are held together by ligaments, which are strong fibrous bands of connective tissue.

The sources of power of this part of your body are the muscles, which are attached to the bones and bring about movement at the joints by contracting and relaxing. The pelvic muscles include the buttock muscles, at the back, which provide strength and support for your hips, spine, and upper body and are especially important during pregnancy. At the base of your pelvis, attached to the area around the outlet, is a sling-like band of muscles that form the pelvic floor. These surround the anus, vagina, and urethra in a double figure-eight pattern. These muscles support all your pelvic and abdominal contents, and your baby passes through them at birth.

The uterus is itself a powerful muscle. It is attached by strong ligaments to the pelvic bones, and is also supported from underneath by the pelvic floor muscles.

Other muscles that are attached to your pelvis are the abdominal, back, and leg muscles. Your pelvis supports and distributes the weight of your upper body, and protects and supports your uterus and growing baby.

Correct tilt of the pelvis during pregnancy is crucial for good posture, for the safe carriage of your child, and for ensuring a good birth. The exercises for pregnancy concentrate on the pelvis and include all the major joints of the body.

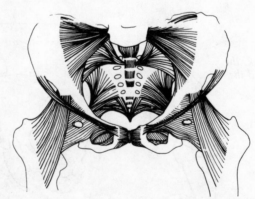

The pelvic ligaments

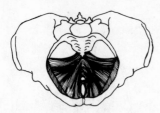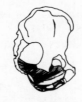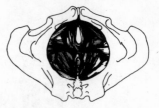

The pelvic floor, as seen from above (left), from the side (center), and from below (right)

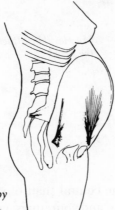

The uterus at full term, attached by strong ligaments to the pelvis

THE SPINE

Your spine is made up of a column of bony vertebrae that extends from the coccyx, or tailbone, at the base; includes the fused vertebrae that make up the sacrum (the back wall of the pelvis); extends to the vertebral column, which begins with the first lumbar vertebra in the lower back; and continues all the way up your back to the smaller vertebrae, which make up the neck and support your head. In the joints between the vertebrae are spongy discs that act as shock absorbers and permit movement of the spine.

With its natural curves, your spine is capable of a range of versatile movements. A healthy spine can bend backwards or forwards; it can twist or go from side to side; and it can combine several of these movements

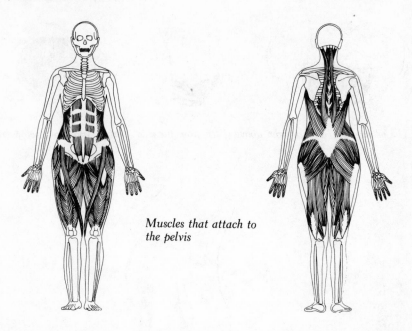

*Muscles that attach to
the pelvis*

in one. Your spine is the central shaft of your skeleton; it supports your
internal organs, your ribs, and your lungs, as well as your head. It contains
your spinal cord, and is thus the supportive structure of your autonomic
nervous system. It controls movement and keeps your body weight balanced. Your spine is dynamic at all times, even when you are asleep.

During pregnancy your spine has the additional task of supporting the
weight of your growing uterus and its contents. As your baby grows, the
natural curves of your spine will adjust to the additional weight in the
front of your body. Most of the stress of this weight is borne by your lower
back, where the weight of your upper body is transferred through your
pelvis down to your legs and feet. After your baby is born your spine will
regain its normal curves and will have to cope with the many hours of
carrying your baby until he or she walks independently.

A healthy spine should adapt easily to the demands of pregnancy and
mothering. However, we are often unaware of underlying imbalances or
stiffness in the spine, and the additional stress of pregnancy may result in
poor posture and back pain. Regularly practicing the exercises in the next
chapter will help to relieve or minimize back pain and will strengthen
your spine and help to maintain its flexibility.

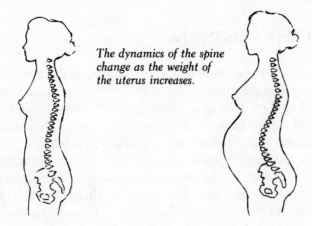

The dynamics of the spine change as the weight of the uterus increases.

THE HEART AND LUNGS

During pregnancy your fluid and blood volume increases considerably to ensure that sufficient blood is pumped to and from the uterus and placenta, as well as the rest of your body. Your heart works harder, and your breathing changes as well. In order to nourish and carry your baby well, your whole body works harder than usual.

As pregnancy advances, the extra weight you are carrying may make it more difficult to exercise and exert yourself in the usual ways. Yet, with birth and motherhood ahead, it is important to maintain or improve your flexibility and strength. Appropriate nonstrenuous exercise will help to keep your cardiovascular system at its best, and ensure that you are breathing well and that the blood going through to your baby is well oxygenated.

Continue with any sport you already play, provided you feel all right about it. Avoid squash, though, as the hard ball could damage your baby. Walking, dancing, and cycling are all suitable. Swimming is particularly beneficial. Try doing your deep breathing (see chapter 4) while swimming the breaststroke.

In pregnancy, lovemaking and orgasm are as beneficial to you as ever, if you enjoy them, and they can't harm your baby. Try different positions—such as all fours, the knee-chest position, and lying side by side like spoons—to avoid any weight on your belly. This is a great time to experiment!

A HEALTHY PREGNANCY

Since your body is well designed to accommodate the physical and emotional changes of pregnancy, you may experience this as a time of great health and vitality. Eating a well-balanced, nutritious diet, getting the right kind of regular exercise, and staying in touch with your feelings will help to ensure your physical and emotional well-being.

However, discomforts such as backache, cramps, constipation, insomnia, and heartburn are common in pregnancy. These can usually be treated with self-help, through exercise or alternative therapies, before they escalate into more serious problems. My book *Natural Pregnancy* (see "Recommended Reading") offers practical guidelines on maintaining your health in pregnancy, and coping with the emotional changes of this time, with a holistic approach aimed to increase self-reliance. The book outlines alternative therapies—such as homeopathy, herbalism, and acupuncture—that can be safely used in pregnancy to enhance your body's natural healing powers. It includes many useful tips on prevention, self-help, and professional treatment of common ailments by natural means.

3 | Yoga-based Exercises for Pregnancy

DURING THE NINE MONTHS OF PREGNANCY YOUR BODY needs to accommodate enormous physiological changes. New demands are placed on your system as you breathe, digest, and excrete—not only for yourself, but also for your growing baby.

In early pregnancy, you are adapting to the hormonal, physical, and psychological upheavals that are common at this time, and you may need to cope with unusual tiredness or nausea. Later on, in mid-pregnancy, you probably feel more settled and enjoy a sense of vitality, health, and well-being. At this time you want to exercise and use your body in a way that makes the most of its transformative potential and is appropriate for pregnancy. In the last few months, as your body adjusts to the increasing weight you are carrying, you can benefit from exercises that protect and strengthen your spine and exercise your whole body without strain. You also need to prepare for the challenges of labor, birth, and motherhood.

Most of the exercises in this chapter are derived from hatha yoga; these are particularly suitable for increasing flexibility during pregnancy. A few are adapted from physical therapy to strengthen certain muscle groups in the body and prevent stress.

Hatha yoga is an ancient system of exercise that originated in paleolithic times in Europe, developed in India, and is now widely practiced all over the world. It is a way to both relax your body and quiet your mind. Most important, yoga, correctly practiced, brings your body into a harmonious balance with the force of gravity, to which our bodies are subject at all times. You can learn, with the help of your breathing and without force or strain of any kind, to let go of unnecessary tension and stiffness in your joints and muscles.

In the preceding chapters, we have seen how the normal physiology of the birth process can best take place when you position your body in harmony with gravity. Each time you practice the exercises recommended in this chapter, you will be developing this instinctive body sense. This will guide you during labor, giving you confidence and faith in your own power. You will be better in touch with your instincts and better able to let go of the fear and tensions that can inhibit the involuntary birth process. It will be easier to accept the change of consciousness and to tolerate the intense sensations that occur as your body opens up to give birth. In the midst of the most tumultuous and painful contractions you will be able to calm yourself by focusing on your breathing, as you will have learned to do in your yoga practice.

Yoga can help you to flow with the challenging transformation of pregnancy and birth. It can bring you greater self-awareness, and it can also increase your awareness of your child's presence inside your body. When you experience the silence within yourself during yoga practice, you will become more aware of the powerful bond between you and your baby. This awareness will enhance your unconscious communication with the baby throughout pregnancy. And by making you more aware of the miracle of creation taking place within and through your body, the exercises can prepare you to love and nourish your baby in the years to come.

HOW DOES YOGA WORK?

Practically speaking, yoga provides a system of exercises to help you recover the natural range of movements your body is designed to make, in harmony with the force of gravity, and to help you maintain structural fitness.

When posture is poor, the body has become "disconnected" from its foundation and has lost its harmonious relationship to gravity. Tension accumulates in the upper body, which becomes top-heavy. Stresses result in pain and disruption of the muscular and skeletal balance, generally accompanied by a psychological feeling of being ungrounded. Hence, rounded shoulders, hunched back, twisted or distorted spine, protruding jaw, shortened neck vertebrae, and stiff legs are all common postural problems that together are a hidden epidemic in our society. Most of us, without being aware of it, end up carrying a load of unnecessary tension, actually bound up in our muscles and joints. This state of affairs is brought about by the stresses and strains of modern life, sedentary lifestyles, loss of contact with nature, poor postural habits and physical education, and the suppression of emotions, all of which are commonplace today.

Yoga gets to the root of tension in the body and gives you an opportunity to release it. Good posture depends on a harmonious balance between your body weight and gravity. Yoga involves first becoming aware of the way your body is supported by and rests on the ground, in whichever posture you assume. For example, if you are standing, you feel your weight dropping downwards onto the floor through your heels (rather like a tree spreading its roots), or, if you are sitting, you feel your pelvis become heavy and the lower part of your spine relax downwards as your weight drops down onto your sitting bones. This is what it means to become "grounded." It gives you a feeling of both physical and psychological stability.

With a secure foundation in the base, your neck, shoulders, and your upper back are well supported, and can thus become light and free. The more firmly your body rests on the ground, the more loose and relaxed it can be above. Like a tree, then, your spine extends in two directions: from the waist down it lengthens towards the Earth, and from the waist up it lengthens towards the sky, as branches and leaves grow towards the light.

Once you have this sense of strong foundation, the next step is to focus on your breathing rhythm. This will help you to still your mind and focus your awareness inwards, to find what I call your "center." Then you can work with the natural "wave" of the breath. You can learn to direct the exhalations mentally downwards, with gravity, towards your "roots," while your inhalations become passive and bring a feeling of lightness upwards from a stable base, thus lengthening the spine. This may sound confusing or odd before you actually try it, but with a bit of practice you can begin to feel how this happens naturally, when your posture is well balanced.

So yoga is not merely about learning various positions. The essence lies in rediscovering your sense of harmonious orientation to the Earth, through focusing on your breathing and the way your body weight balances with the force of gravity. By "grounding" and "centering" yourself through yoga, you can regain a graceful posture and free yourself from tension, pain, and anxiety. This is especially helpful during pregnancy and also continues to be useful when you are in labor and giving birth, without your having to think about it.

Whereas some yoga positions involve a combination of movements that affect different parts of the body simultaneously, a simple forward bend will help us to understand how the underlying mechanical principle of yoga-based exercise works.

A forward bend is a positional exercise to encourage passive relaxation of the hamstring muscles at the back of the legs. In this position the hip joints act as a hinge. As you bend the weight of the trunk falls forward, drawn downwards by gravity until it meets with resistance from the hamstrings. Then the weight of the upper body, helped by gravity, encourages the hamstrings to stretch and lengthen.

Try this:

1. Stand upright with your feet about 12 inches apart and parallel to each other. Allow your weight to settle on your heels as you exhale, until you feel your feet are well grounded. Clasp your hands behind your back.

2. Now, without bending your knees, bend forward slowly from your hips, keeping your arms behind your back and your spine straight.

3. Hold for a few seconds, breathing deeply, and then come up slowly.

You no doubt felt a stretching sensation in the muscles at the back of your legs as the movement caused them to lengthen and relax. If the exercise was painful, you are probably wondering why, if the muscles were relaxing. The reason is your lifestyle so rarely requires such full movements that the hamstring muscles at the back of your legs have shortened and lost their elasticity, restricting your ability to move forward.

Nature has designed your body to be able to fold over like a jackknife, with your belly and chest flat against your thighs and the palms of your hands on the ground in front of you. Of course, during the later months of pregnancy, this can only be done with legs apart to make room for your belly! (See page 74.) In this position your feet are firmly grounded, and gravity draws your trunk forward like a lever from the hips. Your spine should be completely relaxed while the front of your body contracts and the hamstring muscles lengthen and extend. Breathing deeply for a few moments while in the position allows you to release the tightness you feel in your legs and to lengthen and relax your spine, until with practice you can make the movement with greater ease.

You will probably find, as you experiment with other movements, that a state of chronic tension exists throughout your body to some degree, affecting some areas more than others. The most effective way to become more relaxed and supple is by beginning to make the neglected movements we were designed by nature to make. It is simply a matter of spending some time each day practicing them. Gradually stiff muscles will lengthen and regain their elasticity, and joints will become more mobile as tension is released.

The program of yoga-based exercises that follows will cultivate relaxation and flexibility in a safe, unstrenuous way. Pregnancy is a unique and marvelous time to let go of habitual tensions and to allow your body to become more relaxed. If you've never exercised before, you may find some of the positions difficult at first. But gradually, with practice, you'll loosen up.

The Benefits of Yoga-based Exercise

1. As your muscles become more supple and your joints more mobile, the muscular balance that supports and moves your body improves. Muscles work in teams; while one team is relaxing and lengthening, the other is contracting and shortening. When you balance the opposing teams of muscles, your joints articulate better and your posture automatically improves. This ensures that you carry your baby correctly and helps to prevent backache.

2. Breathing well depends on good posture. When your pelvis and spine are in good balance and your shoulders are relaxed, your chest cavity can expand easily so that breathing is unrestricted. This ensures good oxygenation of the blood for you and your baby throughout pregnancy.

3. As you become familiar with the exercises you will find movements that alleviate the minor discomforts of pregnancy, such as heartburn, pain in the hip joints or in the ribs, cramps in the legs, or headaches.

4. Your circulation depends upon your muscles. They act as pumps, making the blood flow through your body and returning the blood to your

heart. If a muscle is tight, then the blood vessels running through it are constricted and your blood circulation (and indeed, indirectly, the circulation to your baby in the womb) is also restricted. The exercises can help to ensure that your baby is getting everything needed to grow healthy and strong. They can also prevent or lessen problems associated with poor circulation—varicose veins, hemorrhoids (piles), and fluid retention. Finally, the exercises tend to lower the blood pressure, and can thus help to prevent problems associated with rising blood pressure (see chapter 7).

5. Yoga-based exercises help to combat fatigue. If muscles are shortened and movement is restricted, the flow of energy is "blocked." After a session of exercise you will feel invigorated and refreshed, and over time this feeling will increase. Your pregnancy can be a time when you feel healthier and more energetic than ever.

6. The most comfortable yoga positions in pregnancy are very similar to positions women instinctively assume in labor. So, by practicing the exercises, you will have cultivated ease and comfort in the natural positions for birth used by women through the ages, without needing to think about it very much. You will be able to move freely and instinctively; your body will know what to do. Yoga will help you to be more deeply in touch with your own center. It will be easier to surrender to the powerful forces within your body during labor.

7. As stiffness lessens, your body becomes free of pain.

8. You will gradually become familiar with the discomforts and even the pain of going beyond your usual limits. As labor and birth will demand going beyond your normal limits of pain endurance, positioning your body to go beyond your normal limits of movement during pregnancy prepares you gradually for this kind of effort. The exercises will teach you to surrender to the forces within your body. This is the best possible practice for labor; it will help you to cope with the intensity of the sensations of your contracting uterus, and will also help to reduce the pain by enabling you to relax and accept the feelings rather than tensing up against them. As one mother said—

> "By exercising, I learned how to be at one physically and emotionally with the changes that would inevitably lead to the birth of my child. The teaching enabled me to 'go with' my body, even when the pain was a burden. I was physically and also mentally prepared for everything that was to happen to me, and I approached the final events with excitement and real confidence."

9. Whatever happens during labor and birth—even if complications arise—practicing yoga-based exercises throughout pregnancy will have been the best way to prepare for a speedy recovery.

THE EXERCISES

Choose a time of day when you have a little time to yourself—first thing in the morning, or perhaps last thing at night. It is best not to eat a large meal beforehand. You will need a carpeted space with one free wall, two pillows, and a low stool or pile of large books.

The exercises are arranged in eight sequences, which include six basic exercises to be practiced daily, or as often as possible (these are marked with asterisks and labeled "Basic" I to VI). The whole program should take about 1½ hours to complete, but you may devise your own personal program concentrating on the basics and then adding others according to preference or need.

For best results, start doing these exercises as early in your pregnancy as possible—any time after the twelfth week, unless your doctor advises you that it is all right to start sooner. However, it is never too late to benefit.

Start off in any easy way, holding each position for as long as you are comfortable, gradually lengthening the time as you become familiar with the movements. Start with a few of the movements, and gradually build up until you are able to go through the full program. The first thing you may feel when you start is your own stiffness, so expect to spend two or three weeks getting to know the exercises. Gradually, as you loosen up, the movements will become pleasurable. You will probably find that some of the movements fit comfortably into your daily habits, that there are some you can practice while watching TV, reading, or talking to friends, and some you would like to concentrate on. Provided you pay careful attention to the instructions and cautions, all the exercises are safe for pregnancy. Once they are familiar to you, you may safely spend longer periods in each position. If any exercise is uncomfortable after you have tried it for a while, then leave it out and concentrate on the others. At first you will find that you can go up to a certain point, and then you begin to feel the stretch. Reach this point and stay with it, breathing deeply, until the stretching sensation eases. Gradually your range of movement will increase, and your body will become more flexible and relaxed.

A Few Words of Warning

You can benefit from yoga whether you have exercised before or not. If, however, you have a chronic back problem or any complication in your pregnancy, such as a history of miscarriage or cervical stitch, then do check with your doctor before exercising, and follow the cautionary notes carefully.

If you begin bleeding at any time in your pregnancy, call your doctor or midwife immediately. Stop exercising, and rest in bed. Although a small amount of bleeding in pregnancy is usually no cause for concern, it could indicate a problem.

Contrary to popular myth, backache should not be an inevitable part of pregnancy. As pregnancy advances, your joints will loosen because of the release of hormones, and your body will need to adapt to the increase in weight. If backache occurs, it is due to postural problems or to an underlying structural imbalance that you may not have been aware of before you became pregnant. If you experience back pain, pain in the sacroiliac joints, tension headaches, sinusitis, or any joint pain, it is advisable to consult a chiropractor, an osteopath, or a physical therapist who specializes in pregnancy (see "Resources").

Practicing these exercises can help to relieve cramps in the calves, backache, varicose veins, hemorrhoids, high blood pressure, sleeplessness, tiredness, nausea, and other common complaints of pregnancy. For best results, however, do read the instructions and cautionary notes carefully before you start each exercise.

If you are carrying a very large baby or twins, these exercises can be invaluable. But do be especially cautious, since your body's systems are all working harder. Listen to any signals your body gives that you should slow down or stop.

Some women find that they are uncomfortable lying on their backs during pregnancy, particularly in the last six weeks. This is because the weight of the heavy uterus presses on the large blood vessels in your abdomen, which slows down your circulation and can cause dizziness. If this happens to you at *any* stage, then roll over onto your side, come up onto your hands and knees, and, in the future, leave out any exercise that involves lying on your back. For most of us, this is no problem, and lying on the back for short periods, provided the knees are bent or the legs up, is very relaxing. However, it is wise for all women to avoid lying on the back during the last six weeks of pregnancy.

Similarly, some women find that the standing positions or forward bends are uncomfortable, or become so if held for too long. At all times, let your body be your guide. Leave out any exercises that don't suit you, and stop to rest when you have had enough.

Useful Tips

- It is important for your well-being and that of your baby that you attend regular prenatal checkups with your midwife, doctor, or clinic as well as do these exercises.
- During your pregnancy, wear flat-heeled shoes. Whenever possible, sit on a low stool or a pile of books instead of on a chair, or sit on the floor cross-legged or with legs apart.
- It is a good idea to get together with another friend who is pregnant, or perhaps a small group, and practice together. Some of the exercises include work with a partner; they are equally beneficial for men, in case your mate wishes to join you.
- It can be very pleasant to precede or follow your stretching session with a warm bath or shower, or perhaps a swim.

Exercise Sequence I: Getting Centered

A. Basic Sitting

Until you are familiar with this exercise it will help if someone reads the instructions aloud very slowly as you do it.

1. Sit with your back supported by a wall. Draw one foot in towards your body, and then place the other comfortably in front of it; or else sit cross-legged. Make sure your sacrum is right up against the wall.

2. Now close your eyes, and release tension in the back of your neck by bringing your chin down a little, towards your chest. Relax your shoulders. Without altering your normal breathing rhythm, focus your awareness on your breathing. As you breathe, become especially aware of the exhalations.

Feel the way your sitting bones contact the floor. With each exhalation, sense your pelvis dropping downwards with gravity, and relax your knees, hips, and legs towards the floor. Release your sacrum downwards so that all of your lower body is well grounded and your back relaxed. Become

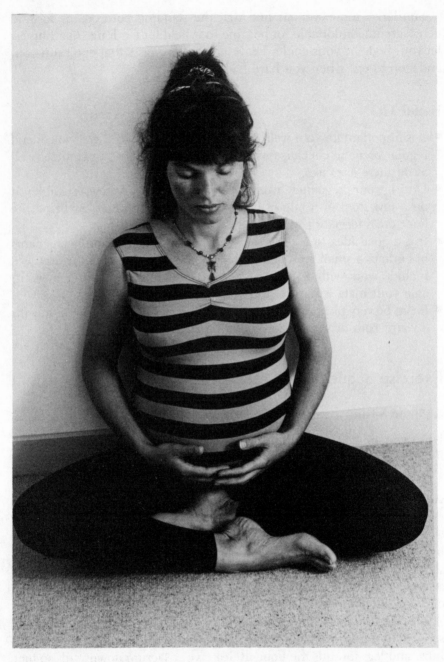

Exercise I A: The basic sitting position

aware of your spine, securely supported from the tailbone upwards, through the lower back, between your shoulders and up into the neck.

With each out-breath relax: release any tension in your eyes, your jaw, your neck and your shoulders, your belly, and your pelvic floor. Place the palms of your hands gently on your lower belly, just above the pubic bone.

B. Breathing (Basic I)*

1. In the basic sitting position, with your awareness still focused on your breathing, begin to pay special attention to the out-breath. Normally we breathe in and out through the nose, but, for now, allow yourself to exhale very slowly through the mouth. When you reach the very end of the exhalation, pause for a moment or two. Then inhale through the nose to gently fill your lungs again.

Continue breathing like this for a few moments, keeping your body completely relaxed. Allow the breath to simply flow at its own pace. The exhalation should be approximately twice as long as the inhalation.

2. Continuing to breathe deeply, out through the mouth and in through the nose, shift your awareness down to your lower belly. See if you can feel the gentle movement of your belly as you breathe. As you exhale, pressure in the abdomen decreases, and your belly should move away from your hands towards your spine. Pause. Then breathe in. As you do, pressure in the abdomen increases, and your belly should expand towards your hands.

Continue breathing like this, feeling your belly contract away from your hands as you breathe out, and expand gently towards your hands as the breath comes in. The rest of your body should remain relaxed and still, with very little movement in the chest and shoulders.

If you find yourself breathing into the chest rather than the belly, as many of us do habitually, keep focusing on your out-breath, and try exaggerating the movement of your belly a little, actually drawing the abdominal muscles away from your hands towards your spine as you exhale, then releasing them towards your hands when you inhale. With a little practice, this movement should become automatic and feel quite natural as your breathing deepens.

3. Make some simple sounds out loud with the exhalation. Start with the sound "ooo" (as in *you*). Feel the sound coming from the very base of the pelvis; continue until the end of the out-breath. Then pause, and

let the in-breath come in as usual. Repeat the sound "ooo" as you breathe out again.

Then try the sound "aaw" (as in *for*), feeling the "aaw" sound coming from the belly, and repeat.

Now try the sound "ah" (as in *far*), coming from the heart or chest.

End up by humming as you exhale.

4. Now place your hands palms up on your knees, and, with your eyes closed and your awareness focused on your breathing, return to your normal breathing, in and out through the nose.

With a partner. Try practicing deep breathing together. Your partner can help by sitting beside you and placing one hand on your lower belly with the other resting gently on your lower back. As you exhale, gentle pressure from your partner's hand in front can remind you to "empty" your belly. As you inhale, breathe in towards your partner's hand.

Benefits. When you breathe deeply you are mainly using your diaphragm muscle, which moves up as you exhale and down as you inhale, creating the fluctuating pressure in the belly. When we are relaxed we naturally breathe abdominally. However, when we become tense or anxious our breathing usually rises and becomes shallow, with most of the movement happening in the chest rather than the belly, and the emphasis on the inhalation rather than the exhalation (see chapter 4).

Practicing deep breathing—

- is calming;
- helps to center you inwardly;
- focuses your awareness on gravity, and thus releases and lengthens the spine;
- helps stretching muscles to release tension and lengthen; and
- thoroughly oxygenates the blood and removes toxins and waste products for both you and your unborn baby.

Breathing with sounds helps to lengthen and deepen your exhalations and also helps you to overcome any inhibition about releasing sound during labor and birth. In labor, releasing sound with the out-breath often helps to reduce the pain of intense contractions. In the expulsive phase, when your baby is being born, making sounds can help to strengthen your pushing efforts.

C. Meditation and Baby Awareness

1. Sit quietly for a few moments and focus your awareness on the rhythm of your breathing. After a while your mind will become quiet as you become more aware of your inner feelings. If thoughts or distractions arise, simply acknowledge them, and then bring your concentration back to the breath.

2. Then focus your awareness on the presence of your baby, sheltered inside you. Imagine for a moment what it must be like for your baby to be inside your womb. Imagine the feeling of the warm amniotic fluid on your baby's skin. Imagine the sounds that your baby can hear: your heart beating day and night, the food moving through your digestive system, the air whooshing through your lungs, and the blood pulsing through the placenta and the umbilical cord. From early pregnancy, and especially in the last few months, your baby can hear the sound of your voice and other sounds from outside, like music or the voices of other family members. He or she may also be sensitive to your thoughts, dreams, and feelings as well as your touch, as you stroke and massage your belly. Allow yourself to become aware of your ability to communicate with your baby, and spend a few more quiet moments together before slowly opening your eyes.

You are now ready to start exercise sequence II.

Exercise Sequence II: Pelvic Release

A. Tailor Pose (Basic II)*

(Caution: In the last weeks of pregnancy, the pubic joint loosens to widen the pelvic outlet for birth. If you feel any pain in this area, do the tailor pose very gently, keeping your feet a comfortable distance from your body and avoiding any strain. Do not hold for more than three minutes. You can practice this daily, if it helps; otherwise, leave the position out altogether.)

1. Sit against a wall, with your lower back supported by the wall. Bend your knees, and place the soles of your feet together, with the outside edges touching and the soles opening out like the pages of a book.

2. Hold your feet with your hands, and stretch up and lengthen your

spine for a moment. Now let go of your feet, and allow your knees to relax towards the floor.

Breathe comfortably and deeply. With each exhalation, feel how your sitting bones contact the floor, and release your lower back and pelvis downwards with gravity. With each inhalation, feel your spine become longer and lighter, remembering to keep your shoulders, head, and neck relaxed and your pelvis grounded.

Feel your hip joints relax, tension melting towards the floor, allowing your pelvis to feel more and more grounded as the upper body loosens. Hold for a few moments, releasing tension and opening into the posture with your breathing.

With a partner. Sit in the tailor pose with your partner sitting behind

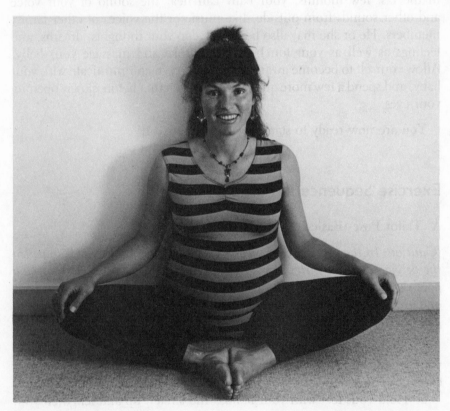

Exercise II A: Tailor pose

you. Let your partner support your spine by placing the soles of both feet against your lower back or, alternatively, one foot above the other along your spine. This will prevent your pelvis from tilting backwards and your spine from "collapsing."

Hold for a few moments.

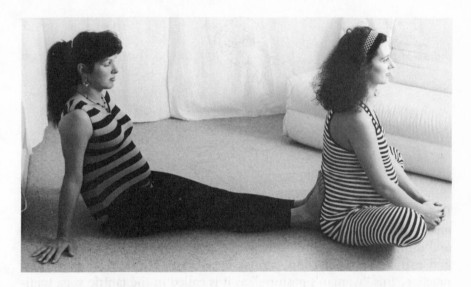

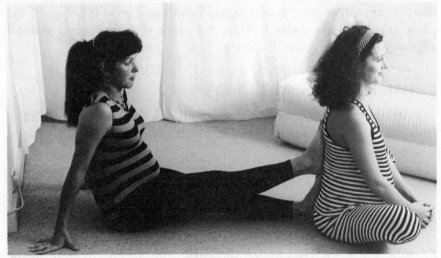

Tailor pose with partner

Advanced posture. If your legs are resting on the floor, hold your feet, and, with your spine free, lean forward from the hips, keeping your pelvis in full contact with the floor. Lean only as far forward as you can without bending your back. If the forward movement is easy, then place your hands palms down on the floor in front of you, and extend your trunk forward from the hips as far as your belly will comfortably allow.

Advanced tailor pose

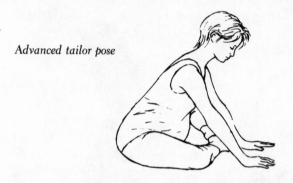

Benefits. This exercise releases tension in the hips, groin, knees, and ankles, and helps to widen the pelvic diameters. It relaxes the pelvic floor and improves circulation to the whole area. It should be practiced daily and can be used for short periods as a sitting position. With regular practice, this "woman's posture," as it is called in the tantric yoga tradition, is said to promote gynecological health and good function of the pelvic organs. It also helps to bring the pelvis into a balanced postural alignment with the rest of the body.

B. Ankle Release

1. From the tailor pose, straighten your legs out together in front of you, and extend your heels. Feel the stretch along the backs of your legs, and then point your toes.

Repeat 20 times, alternately extending your heels and pointing your toes.

2. Separate your legs a little, and rotate your ankles in full circles, first inwards and then outwards. Do 20 each way.

Benefits. These exercises loosen the ankles, improve movement in the joints, and reduce swelling.

C. Knee Bend

1. Now bend your right knee and, with your left leg still extended, place your right foot on the left thigh, bringing it up towards the groin as far as you can comfortably manage.

2. Extend your left heel, feeling the back of your left leg contact the floor. Place your right hand on your right knee and breathe deeply. Feel your weight settle towards the floor with each exhalation, and feel both sitting bones contact the floor. Hold for a few moments.

3. Repeat on the other side, extending your right leg and bending the left. Hold for a few moments.

4. Release the left leg, bend the knees, and place both feet together again in tailor pose.

Benefits. This exercise will help to reduce stiffness in the knees, hips, and ankles.

Exercise II C: Knee bend

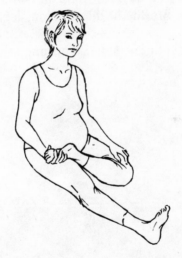

D. Legs Wide Apart

1. Making sure your lower back is still in contact with the wall, spread your legs apart as wide as possible. At first, let your legs feel heavy and floppy. It helps to massage your thighs with your hands. Breathe deeply, grounding your pelvis with each exhalation.

2. Keeping your thighs relaxed and heavy, slowly extend your heels and stretch your calf muscles so the backs of your knees move down towards the floor.

3. Hold for up to three minutes, breathing deeply. As you exhale, feel your weight settle into your pelvis and the backs of your legs. Allow your spine and upper body to lengthen and lighten with each in-breath, keeping your neck and shoulders relaxed.

With a partner. Sit with your legs wide apart and your partner behind you. Your partner should support your spine by placing the soles of both feet against your lower back, or one foot above the other along your spine, as for the tailor pose. Hold for up to three minutes.

Advanced Posture. If you are able to, lean forward gently from the hip, with your palms or even your elbows on the floor (or hold your ankles). Keep your spine loose and free, your pelvis grounded, and your neck and shoulders relaxed. Lean as far as you can comfortably manage without bending your back. Breathe in this position, lengthening and loosening your spine.

End by bending your knees and returning to the tailor pose.

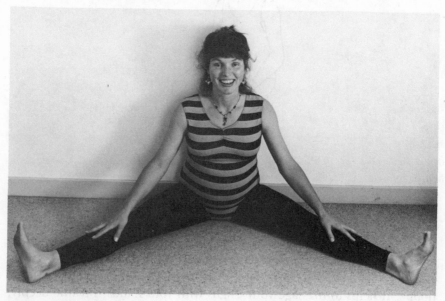

Exercise II D: Legs wide apart

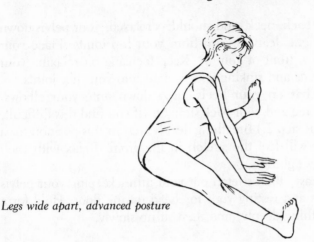

Legs wide apart, advanced posture

Benefits. This exercise widens the pelvis while releasing tension in the hamstring muscles at the backs of the legs. It relaxes the pelvic floor and grounds the lower body, encouraging the release of tension in the spine, neck, and shoulders. It also increases mobility of the hip joints.

Exercise Sequence III: Kneeling Positions

(Caution: If the kneeling positions cause discomfort in your ankles, then place one or two cushions underneath your buttocks. This will reduce pressure from your weight on your calves and ankles. A firm bolster-shaped cushion is ideal for this; if you have one, place it lengthwise between your knees, as you would sit astride a horse. Foot cramps in the kneeling positions—"beginner's cramps," I call them—will pass with practice.)

A. Kneeling with Knees Wide Apart (Basic III)*

1. Kneel on the floor with your pelvis resting on your heels, your knees as wide apart as possible, and your toes pointing inwards towards each other (*a*). With your awareness on your breathing, exhale, and relax your lower back downwards towards your feet, so your pelvis drops down onto your heels.

2. Keeping your back, neck, and shoulders relaxed, your pelvis down and your spine straight, lean forward from your hip joints. Place your palms on the floor in front of you (*b*). Keep focusing on relaxing your lower back downwards and sinking your weight into your hip joints.

3. With your pelvis on your heels, drop down onto your elbows, keeping your spine free and your back straight. (If you find this difficult, then only go as far as step 2.) Breathing deeply, rest in this position for a few moments. You will feel the stretch in the groin. Relax with each exhalation, releasing tightness.

4. If step 3 was easy, then stretch out your arms, keeping your pelvis down on your heels and resting your forehead on the floor. Hold for a few moments, breathing deeply, and then sit up slowly.

With a Partner. Your partner can help by placing one hand on your sacrum and gently leaning his or her body weight downwards to anchor your pelvis. Let your partner know how much pressure is comfortable.

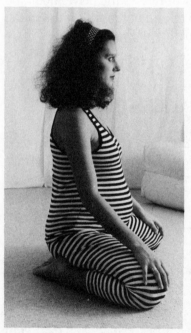
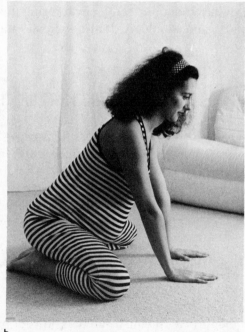

a   b

Exercise III A: Kneeling with knees wide apart

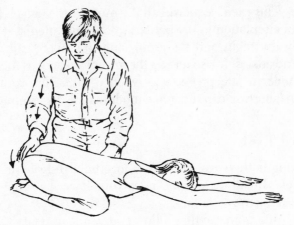

Exercise III A, with a partner

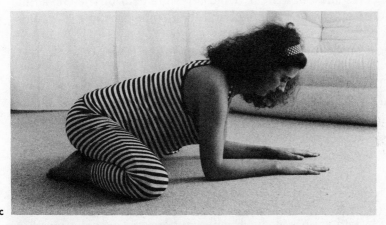

c

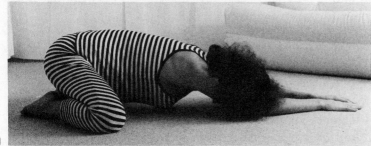

d

Benefits. This exercise relaxes all the muscles that attach to the pelvis and improves circulation to the pelvic area and the uterus. It releases tension in the inner thighs and the groin, and improves flexibility of the hips, knees, and ankles. It also relaxes the lower back, and is therefore especially comfortable in late pregnancy, when it takes the extra weight off the spine. In labor you can use it in a modified way by leaning over a cushion.

B. Spinal Twist

1. Bring both knees and ankles together, and sit with your pelvis on your heels. Breathing deeply, relax your lower back down towards your heels with each exhalation.
2. Starting from the hips, allow your spine to rotate gently to the right as you breathe out. Move your left hand across your body and hold on to your right thigh as you turn.
Without leaning back, continue gently to rotate the spine, looking around over your right shoulder to include the vertebrae of the neck. Close your eyes and relax them. Hold for a moment or two, breathing deeply and dropping your tailbone, and then come back to the "center" for a moment.
3. Repeat on the other side. Come back to the center.

Benefits. Twisting stimulates the natural lubrication of the spinal joints and promotes flexibility and strength of the spinal column. It improves circulation of the cerebrospinal fluid and thus nourishes the whole nervous system. It also releases tension in the oblique muscles of the trunk and gently stretches the strong ligaments that support the uterus.

C. Pelvic Lift

1. Start by sitting on your heels with your knees and ankles together. Drop your chin forward towards your chest, and lean back onto your hands.
2. Keeping your head forward and knees together, inhale and tuck in your sacrum, lengthening the base of your spine. Gently lift your pelvis upwards so that you feel the stretch along the front of the thighs.
3. Hold for a few seconds, then relax with the exhalation, dropping your pelvis back onto your heels.
4. Repeat four or five times.

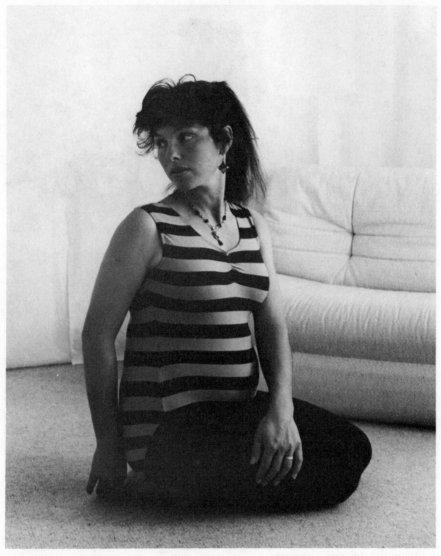

Exercise III B: Spinal twist

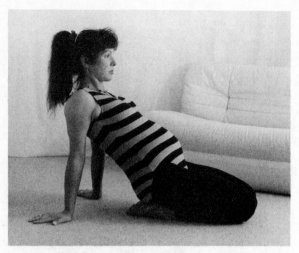

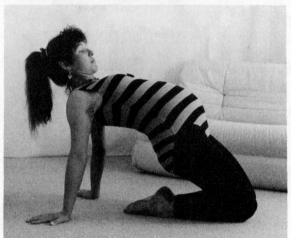

Exercise III C: Pelvic lift

Benefits. This exercise strengthens the lower back and stretches and strengthens the front of the thighs. It can reduce or prevent backache or pain in the sacroiliac joints.

D. All Fours Tuck-in

1. Come forward onto your hands and knees, placing both your palms and your knees about 12 inches apart. Drop your tailbone, and tuck your pelvis under, arching your lower back.

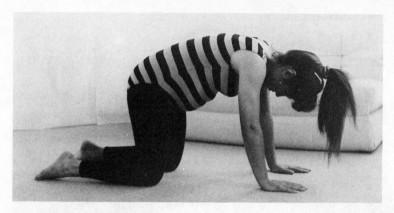

Exercise III D: All fours tuck-in

Release gently, coming back to the horizontal. Avoid releasing too far into a sway-backed position.

2. Repeat several times.

Benefits. This will strengthen your lower back and alleviate backache.

E. Movements for Labor

1. Still on all fours, try rolling your hips around in wide circles, breathing deeply and focusing on your exhalations (*a*). Continue for a few moments, breathing out and letting go, and then reverse and circle in the opposite direction.

2. Rock gently backwards and forwards, exhaling as your weight moves towards your heels, inhaling as it moves onto your hands.

3. Raise yourself to an upright kneeling position, and roll your hips some more (*b*). Bring one knee up, so you are in a half-kneeling and half-squatting position. Rock backwards and forwards with each breath (*c*).

4. Stand up, and place your feet parallel, about 12 inches apart, your hands on your hips and knees slightly bent. Roll your hips in both directions alternately, focusing on breathing out and letting go. Keeping your upper body relatively still, let your pelvis rotate like a belly dancer.

Benefits. This is good practice for labor, when rolling the hips helps to dissipate the pain during contractions, enhances dilation of the cervix, and assists the baby's journey through the pelvic canal.

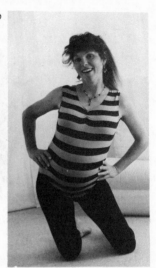

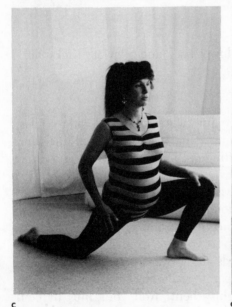

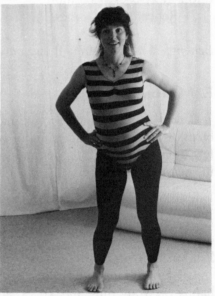

Exercise III E: Movements for labor

Exercise Sequence IV: Reclining Positions

(Caution: Towards the end of pregnancy, when your belly becomes heavy, you may want to avoid lying on your back when you exercise or sleep. This is to ensure that the weight of your belly does not compress the large blood vessels that supply the uterus and baby with oxygen and nutrients and remove waste products. From the beginning of the thirty-fourth week of your pregnancy, or at any stage of pregnancy when you feel uncomfortable or dizzy lying on your back, leave out this sequence of exercises. If you are comfortable on you back, however, the exercises will be relaxing and enjoyable, allowing complete release of tension in your spine, until six weeks before your due date.)

A. Abdominal Toner

1. Lie on your back with your knees bent and the soles of your feet touching the wall. Place your feet parallel and about 12 inches apart. Clasp your hands behind your head, and place your elbows on the floor (*a*). This is the resting position.

Breathe deeply into your belly, and relax your shoulders, spine, and lower back onto the floor. With each exhalation, drop the back of your

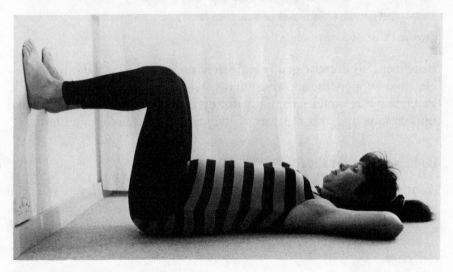

Exercise IV A: Abdominal toner (a)

waist downwards. Feel your abdominal muscles tighten, and your belly move downwards, as you exhale. Feel your muscles relax, and your belly gently rise, as you inhale.

2. Now, with an exhalation, lift your head and arms off the floor towards your feet (*b*). Hold for a second, inhale, and then exhale and return to the resting position. Take a breath in and out.

3. Repeat six times, then relax.

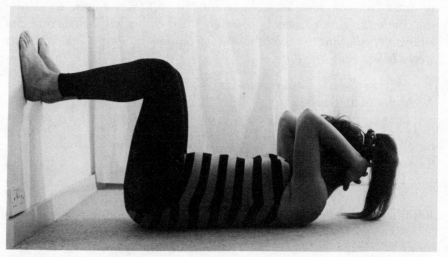

Exercise IV A: Abdominal toner (b)

Benefits. This exercise gently and safely strengthens the abdominal muscles that support the growing uterus, while protecting the lower back. Practicing this exercise regularly during pregnancy maintains abdominal muscle tone and aids recovery of the abdominal muscles after birth.

B. Legs Apart on the Wall (Basic IV)*

(*Caution: This exercise can be practiced up until six weeks before your due date, when you should concentrate on the sitting version of this exercise [II D] instead. If you feel dizzy or uncomfortable when lying on your back at any stage of your pregnancy, then leave out all exercises in this position [see page 63].*)

1. Sit alongside a wall with your hip touching the wall. Swing around so your legs extend up the wall and you are lying on your back (*a*). Your trunk should be at a 90-degree angle to your legs; your buttocks should touch the wall.

Relax and breathe deeply, your belly moving gently inward towards your spine as you exhale and outward as you inhale. Feel the back of your waist contact the floor; relax your shoulders, bringing them down towards your pelvis and spreading them wide onto the floor. Tuck in your chin to lengthen and relax the back of your neck, and release any tension in your jaw and around your eyes.

2. With your awareness on the backs of your legs, stretch your calves and extend your heels. As you exhale, allow your legs to open as wide as possible (*b*). You will feel the stretch in the inner thighs. Keep breathing deeply, dropping the back of your waist, with your knees straight. Hold for only a few seconds the first time you try this. Gradually extend the time to three minutes as tension eases.

3. Bend your knees, and bring the soles of your feet together, close to your body. With your hands, gently bring your knees closer to the wall (*c*).

4. Alternate steps 2 and 3, repeating several times.

Benefits. One of the most beneficial exercises, this releases tension from the adductors, or large muscles of the inner thighs. These have an important influence on the genital area. Relaxing the inner thighs releases blocked sexual energy, improving orgasmic release in lovemaking and making it easier to let go during birth. The exercise relaxes the pelvic floor, and, by preparing you both physically and psychologically to open your body, it can help to reduce inhibition and fear. It also allows complete relaxation of the spine.

This exercise can be practiced daily throughout pregnancy. At first it may seem rather difficult, but after a week or two of regular practice you will find it deeply relaxing and invigorating. Practiced last thing at night after a warm bath, it will help to prevent insomnia and discomfort in bed. Practiced twice daily for up to three minutes, it will help with varicose veins by helping the blood flow from the feet down the legs to the thighs.

With a partner. While you lie on your back with your legs extended vertically up the wall, have your partner follow these instructions:

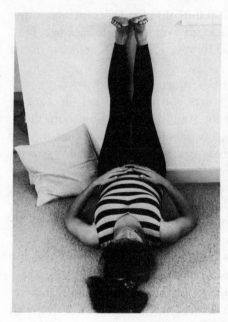
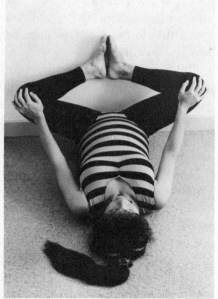
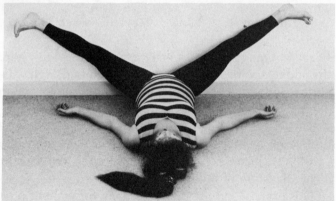

Exercise IV B: Legs apart on the wall (a, b, *and* c)

1. Sitting comfortably behind her head, place your palms on her shoulders, and lean forward to press her shoulders gently down and towards the wall to relax them (*a*). Hold for a few seconds, and then release.

2. Lift her head up, supporting the base of the skull. Encourage her to trust you, to relax and let go. Then massage, firmly but gently, from

the base of the neck towards you, with even strokes (*b*). Alternating your hands, continue until you feel the back of her neck relax and lengthen.

3. Place her head gently down, pulling softly towards you at the same time, so the back of the neck stays as long as possible.

4. Gently place your palms on her forehead, and rest your fingertips on top of the eyelids (*c*). Relax and breathe deeply for a few moments, allowing her to relax and release any tension around her eyes.

5. Hold her gently by the wrists from underneath, and lean back, exerting a firm but gentle traction on the shoulders (*d*). This helps to create more space for the baby and relaxes the upper back and rib cage. Hold for a few seconds, and then gently release her arms to the floor.

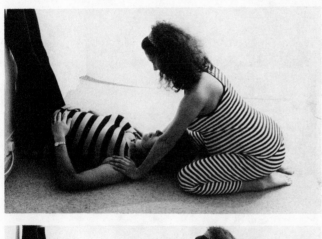

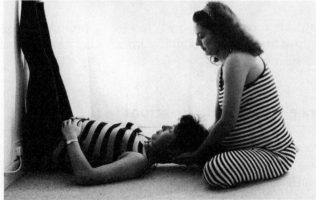

Exercise IV B, with a partner (a *and* b)

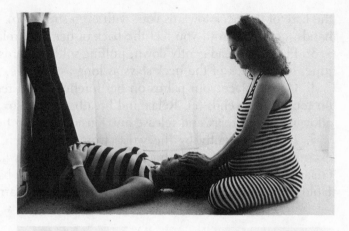

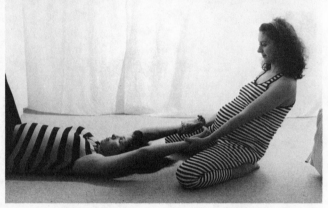

Exercise IV B, with a partner (c *and* d)

Roll over onto your side and come up slowly to a sitting position. Allow your circulation to adjust to sitting for about five minutes before you stand up to progress to the next exercise.

Exercise Sequence V: Standing Positions

(Caution: A few women feel lightheaded when standing for any length of time during pregnancy. If this happens to you, omit this sequence or do it very gently, holding only for short intervals and resting on all fours between exercises.)

A. Basic Standing Position

1. Stand with your feet about 12 inches apart. Turn your heels out slightly so that the outside edges of your feet are parallel.

2. Now press your big toe down onto the floor, and spread your feet out wide by stretching and separating your toes. Feel the way the soles of your feet contact the ground. Bring your weight to rest evenly on both legs.

3. Breathe evenly, in and out through the nose. As you exhale, feel your weight dropping down into your heels, so that each exhalation makes you feel more and more grounded, like a tree growing deeper and deeper roots. Lift your arches so your weight is supported by your heels, the outside edges of your feet, and your toes.

4. Now, with your feet firmly planted, relax your knees, and drop your sacrum and tailbone so your pelvis tucks under gently to support your upper body. Relax your shoulders and neck, and be aware of your head balanced evenly on top of the neck vertebrae. Lengthen the back of your neck by bringing your chin forward. Remember that you are like a tree: from the waist your spine extends down towards the ground; from the waist up it lengthens and extends up towards the sky.

Benefits. Most people habitually turn the heels in, and the toes out, when they stand and walk. This makes the bones of the leg rotate outwards and can create stress and pressure in the knee and hip joints. In many cases this is a cause of sacroiliac pain or backache in pregnancy. By instead turning the heels out slightly so the outside edges of the feet are

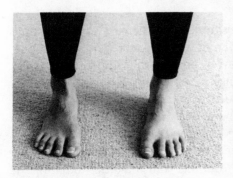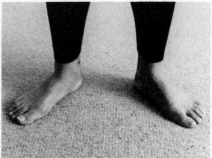

Exercise V A: Correct foot position (left); incorrect foot position (right)

parallel, you position the feet correctly in relation to the knee and hip joints so your lower back widens and your body weight is transferred without stress from the trunk to the ground.

The basic standing position in yoga, or "Mountain Pose," forms the foundation for good posture. As the name implies, the position promotes calmness, balance, strength, and stability. If you make sure that your feet are parallel, your heels well grounded, and your tailbone dropped when you stand or walk, you will minimize stress on your lower back, thus helping to prevent back pain and sciatic pain. Awareness of the way you stand is the key to graceful posture in pregnancy.

B. Warm Up

If you prefer, do this exercise while sitting or kneeling instead of standing.

1. In the basic standing position, roll your head around very slowly, like a big, soft, heavy ball, to release tension in the neck. Pause and breathe for a few seconds if you feel any pain, allowing the tension to release before you continue. Breathe evenly and gently, and relax your jaw. Move only your head and neck to make a complete circle. Repeat several times.

2. Reverse and roll several times in the other direction. Come back to the center.

3. Now roll your shoulders only, first forward and then backward, several times in each direction.

C. Pregnancy Sun Salute

1. Stand in the basic standing position. Place the palms of your hands together in the prayer position an inch or two in front of your breastbone, fingers pointing up, elbows out, so your arms form a horizontal line (a). Relax, and focus on your breathing, dropping your weight from your lower back down into your heels. Inhale.

2. Now exhale, and bring your hands down to form the bottom of an imaginary circle, palms down, fingertips touching (b).

3. Inhaling, bring your arms up slowly as if you were drawing a big wide circle, then place your palms together, your fingertips touching the top of the circle (c).

4. Exhaling, bend forward slowly (d). Gently relax your upper body

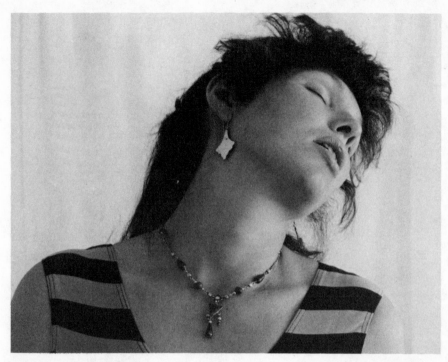

Exercise V B: Head roll

completely, letting your arms, head, and neck hang forward loosely (*e*). Stay in this forward-bend position for one more inhalation and long exhalation, dropping your weight into your heels and feeling the stretch at the back of the legs (*f*).

5. Inhale, and begin to come up slowly, uncurling your spine from the base. Lift your arms as if you were pulling an imaginary piece of string up from between your feet to the top of the circle, at arms length above your head (*g*).

6. With your shoulders relaxed, place your palms together (*h*).

7. Exhale, and bring the arms down in a wide circle (*i*).

As you inhale, return to the prayer position, with palms together (*j*). Exhale, and lengthen your lower back downwards with your weight dropping toward the floor through your heels.

8. With the next inhalation, begin the cycle again. Repeat about four times, breathing with your movements but stopping as soon as you feel you have had enough.

a–e

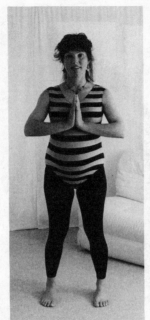
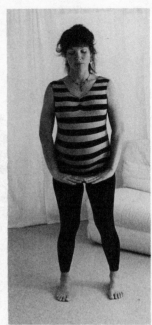

f–j

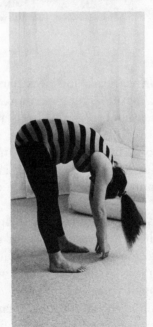
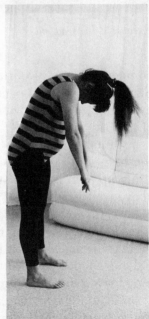

Exercise V C: Pregnancy
sun salute

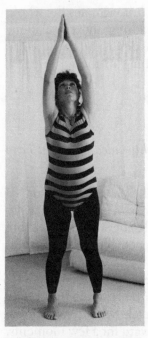
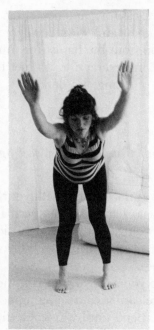
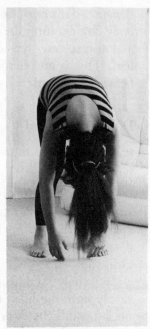
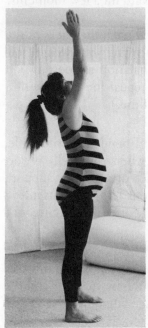
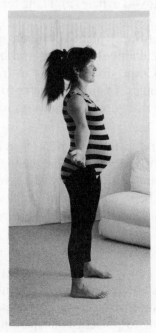
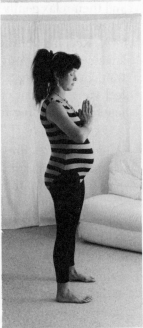

Benefits. This exercise is calming and centering. It invigorates the whole body, by opening the chest and stimulating breathing and circulation, and also releases tension from the hamstring muscles at the backs of the legs. This is an energizing exercise to do first thing in the morning or between long intervals of sitting at a desk.

D. Forward Bend

(Caution: Leave this out if it makes you feel lightheaded or if you have severe hemorrhoids.)

1. On a nonslippery surface, stand with your feet 2 to 3 feet apart. (If you have a nonslip yoga mat, you may wish to place your feet wider apart.) Turn your heels out slightly so the outside edges of your feet are parallel, and bring your weight onto the outside edges, lifting your arches. Grip well with your toes.

2. Exhale, and drop your weight into your heels. Then bend forward slowly from the hips, releasing your spine, upper body, arms, head, and neck towards the floor. Bend until you feel a stretch behind your knees, and then relax gently as you exhale (*a*). Hang forward for a few moments, breathing deeply.

3. Keeping your feet firmly planted, stretch and open the backs of the knees, pointing your tailbone downwards and bringing your weight forward over your toes. Come up slowly on an inhalation as soon as you feel you have had enough. (You may prefer to repeat the movement a few times, holding for only a few seconds each time.)

Alternative Posture. If you find the basic forward bend uncomfortable, particularly towards the end of your pregnancy when your belly is very heavy, place your hands on a windowsill, table, or chair for support, forming a right angle between your trunk and your legs (*b*). This allows the spine to relax and lengthen while well supported in a horizontal position.

Benefits. The forward bend relaxes and lengthens the hamstring muscles at the backs of the legs and releases tension from the pelvic floor and the spine. It also helps to improve circulation and lessen fatigue, and it relaxes the bowel, thus helping to prevent constipation.

a

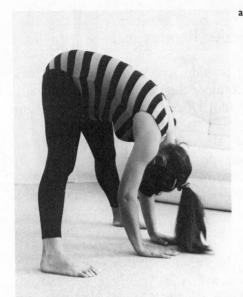

Exercise V D: Forward bend

b

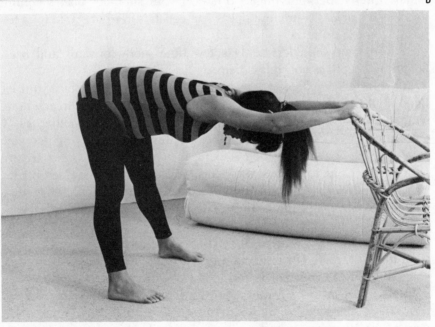

Exercise Sequence VI: Shoulder Release

1. Stand in the basic standing position with heels and lower back releasing downwards. (If standing is uncomfortable, sit or kneel instead.) Breathe deeply for a few moments, and, with each exhalation, allow your shoulders to drop.

Keeping your heels and lower back down, raise your arms gently above your head without tensing or lifting your shoulders. If you do this correctly, you will sense the back of the rib cage staying down rather than lifting. Clasp two fingers of one hand with the other and breathe easily, exhaling down through your ribs, sacrum, and heels towards the floor (*a*).

Lower your arms slowly.

2. Now bring your arms gently backwards, relaxing your shoulders, ribs, sacrum, and heels downwards with each breath, and clasp your hands, interlacing your fingers (*b*). Feel your shoulder blades coming together in back as your chest opens and expands in front. Hold for a few breaths, and then relax.

3. Roll your shoulders softly a few times both forwards and back, breathing deeply as you relax them.

Put your left arm behind you, bending your elbow, and place your left hand up the middle of your back. Raise your right arm, and reach down with your right hand to clasp the fingers of both hands together (*c*). (If your fingers won't meet, use a soft belt as illustrated [*d*].) Lengthen your lower back downwards, gently tucking in your pelvis to avoid arching your back. Hold for a few moments, relaxing your shoulder blades, sacrum, and heels downwards with each exhalation. Your right elbow should be pointing at the ceiling, your left elbow to the floor. Relax.

Repeat on the other side.

4. Kneel facing a wall, with your knees wide apart about 12 inches from the wall, and your buttocks on your heels. Breathe deeply, and, as you exhale, relax your pelvis and thighs downwards.

Stretch your arms up gently over your head, and place your palms on the wall at shoulder's width apart, spreading your fingers. Tuck under your pelvis so your sacrum drops towards your heels and your lower back remains relaxed. Keep your palms as high as possible and your elbows straight, if you can (*e*). Each time you breathe out, relax your chest towards the floor without moving your hands. Concentrate on keeping

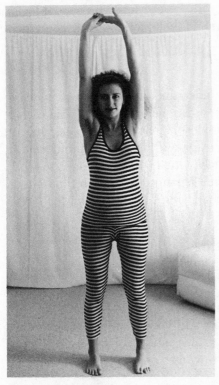

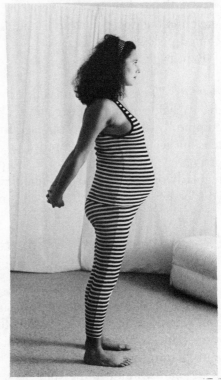

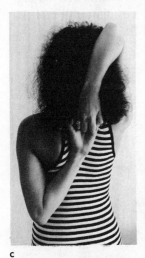

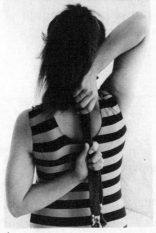

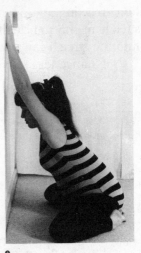

Exercise VI: Shoulder release

your tailbone down to avoid arching your lower back. You should feel a stretch in the upper arms and shoulders. Hold for a few breaths, and then come up slowly.

Repeat once or twice.

Benefits. These exercises relax the shoulders and the rib cage and increase the capacity of the chest cavity. They can help relieve the pain that commonly occurs in the rib cage in late pregnancy, relieve or prevent tension headaches, and improve breathing and posture. Although most pregnancy exercises emphasize the pelvic area, it is important to work regularly on the shoulders to maintain a balanced relaxation throughout your body and to strengthen them for carrying your baby after the birth.

Exercise Sequence VII: Squatting

A. Calf Stretch

1. Stand facing the wall. Place your left leg in front of your right, with both feet pointing directly towards the wall. Bend your left knee; keep your right knee straight. Clasp your hands, and lean forward, placing your elbows and forearms on the wall. Move your right foot back as far as you can without lifting your heel.

Breathing deeply, sink your right heel onto the floor with each exhalation, relaxing and opening the back of the right knee. You will feel the stretch in the right calf muscle and along the achilles tendon. Breathe into the stretch for a while.

2. Change legs. Repeat two or three times on both legs.

CRAMPS

When seized by leg cramps, extend your heel, bringing your toes towards your body, and massage the muscle gently. No one knows for sure what causes leg cramps in pregnancy, but the calf stretch, combined with plenty of general exercise, usually helps to lessen or eradicate them. Calcium supplements may be helpful (make sure these are combined with magnesium and are lead-free.)

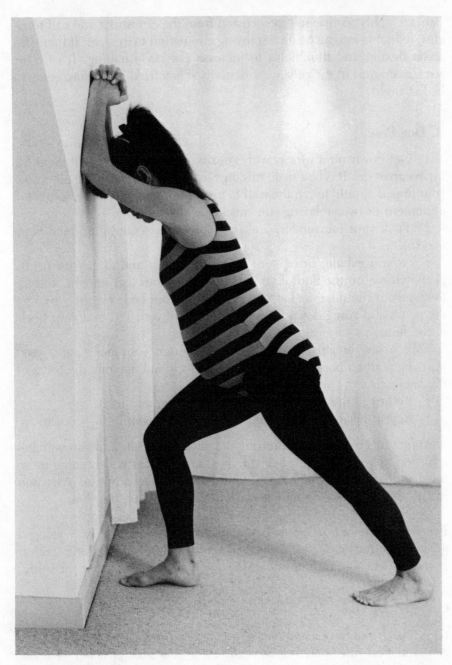

Exercise VII A: Calf stretch

Benefits. This posture releases tension from the hamstring and calf muscles, reducing fatigue while improving circulation to the legs. It increases ankle flexion and thus helps to increase ease in squatting. It eases or reduces cramps in the calves, particularly if practiced just before going to bed at night.

B. Dog Pose

1. Get down on all fours with your hands and knees both about 12 inches apart (*a*). It is best to do this on a firm, nonslip yoga mat; otherwise your fingers should touch the wall to prevent slipping. Breathe deeply for a moment or two, relaxing your neck and shoulders.

2. Tuck your toes under, and lift your pelvis, coming up onto your toes (*b*).

3. As you exhale, bring your pelvis backwards and drop your heels, placing them on the floor if you can (*c*). Keep your legs straight, and try to keep your shoulders and arms relaxed, with your body weight bypassing the pelvis and going down through the back of your legs and your heels to the floor.

Take a few breaths, exhaling down through your heels, and keep bringing your tailbone back towards your heels and opening the backs of the knees.

4. Return to the resting position on all fours, and relax.

5. Repeat twice more, holding for short periods only, if you want.

At first this exercise will probably be rather difficult, and you will feel a bit top-heavy. With practice, the backs of the legs will become more open and less tense, and you will find it easier to feel a release of tension in the shoulders and spine when the heels can touch the floor.

Benefits. Same as for the calf stretch. Also, once you have developed greater ease in the dog pose you will find it helpful in releasing tension from the neck and shoulders and in stretching and elongating the spine.

C. Squatting (Basic V)*

(Caution: If you have hemorrhoids [piles], varicosities, or a cervical stitch, or if you find full squatting difficult, use a low stool or a pile of books whenever you practice squatting [a]. *Start squatting with a partner [see*

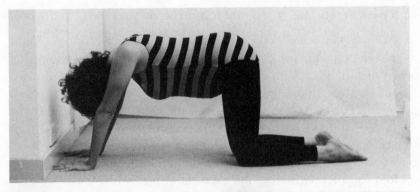

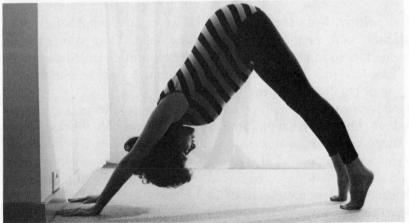

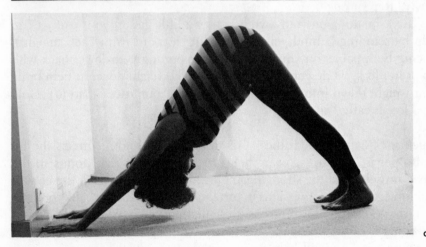

Exercise VII B: Dog pose

"With a partner," below] if you find it difficult on your own, or else hold onto something firm like a window ledge or the edge of your bathtub.)

1. To squat on your own, place your feet 18 inches apart and parallel or turned out slightly. With your heels flat, bend your knees, and place your hands on the floor, then drop your pelvis between your legs and clasp your hands. Separate your knees with your elbows, and lift the arches of your feet (*b*). Keep your shoulders and spine relaxed and your tailbone dropped towards your heels. You may find it helpful to squat close to a wall with just your sacrum touching for support.

2. Hold for a few minutes, and then stand up.

With a partner. Hold each other by the wrists, and stand a full arm's length away from each other with elbows straight. Your partner should place one foot in front of the other, with heels firmly planted and pelvis tucked under, and lean back slightly to support your weight without straining or bending his or her back.

Stand with your feet about 18 inches apart and parallel or only slightly turned out. On an exhalation, drop your heels down onto the floor, bend your knees, and bring your pelvis down between your knees, holding onto your partner for support. Lift your arches, bringing your weight onto the outside edges of your feet, and spread your knees as wide as possible (*c*). With each exhalation, relax your shoulders and spine and drop your tailbone towards your heels. Hold for a few breaths, and then stand up slowly. Repeat once.

When squatting on your own becomes a little easier, your partner can help by standing behind you and bending forward (with back straight), placing both palms on your knees and supporting your lower back with his or her legs, while gently leaning her body weight down to help bring your weight down into your heels and spread your knees apart (*d*). Hold for a few breaths, and relax.

Benefits. Squatting opens the pelvis to its widest. It also corrects the tilt of the pelvis, and in this way helps to produce the right tonus in the pelvic muscles and the strong ligaments to hold the uterus in the correct position against the spine. This in turn helps to position the baby correctly for birth. Squatting also improves circulation to the whole pelvic area, prevents or eases constipation, and relaxes the pelvic floor. Practicing squatting regularly will help you to develop ease in the position so you

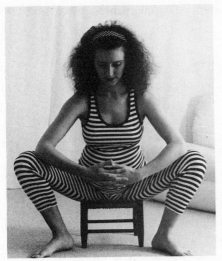

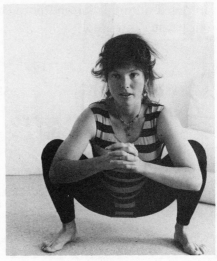

a

b

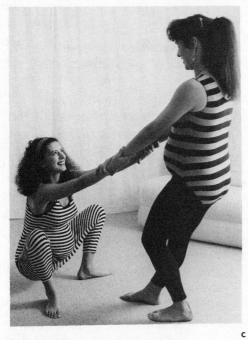

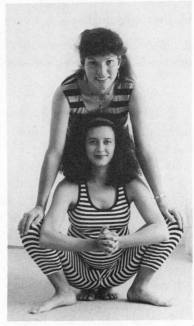

c

d

Exercise VII C: Squatting

can use it during labor and birth (when you may also be supported by your partner or a stool).

CONSTIPATION

Besides squatting, eating bran and dried fruit helps relieve constipation. Make sure that you are taking enough fluids and that your diet contains plenty of vegetables, raw fruit, and salads. All grains should be whole, as refined grains tend to be very constipating. Make sure you act on the urge to defecate when you feel it, for delay could cause constipation. You might place a low stool on either side of the toilet for your feet. This allows you to defecate in more of a squatting position, which relaxes the bowel. Walking and exercising daily are also important.

D. Pelvic Floor Exercise (Basic VI)*

(Caution: If you have hemorrhoids, vulval varicosities, or a cervical stitch, use the knee-chest position [page 131] instead of squatting.)

1. Squat on your toes, your hands on the floor in front of you.
2. Close your eyes and focus your awareness on your pelvic floor—the sling of muscles that surround your urethra, vagina, and anus and form the base of your pelvis. Your baby will pass through the vaginal muscles when you give birth.
3. As you inhale, draw your pelvic floor muscles upwards towards your uterus, contract them, and hold for a moment.
Exhale and relax. Repeat several times.
4. Now inhale and draw the pelvic floor up. Hold the muscles tight while you exhale, then inhale again, still holding, and finally release your breath and the pelvic floor together in four little stages with a long release at the end.
Repeat twice. This will become easier with practice.
5. Now tighten and let go quickly about ten times while breathing normally. (If you have hemorrhoids or vulval varicosities, try doing this in the knee-chest position 50 to 100 times every morning and evening to improve muscle tone and reduce varicosities.)

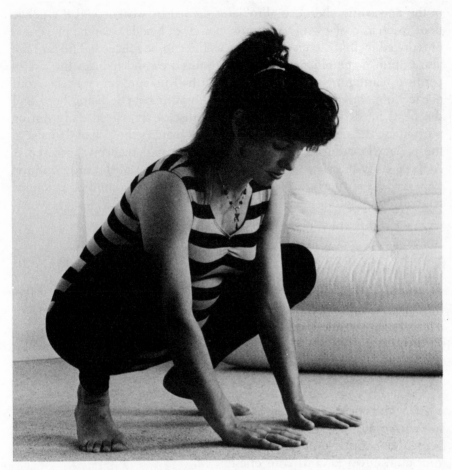

Exercise VII D: Pelvic floor exercise

Especially in the last weeks before the birth, you might occasionally visualize the baby's head coming down and emerging from your pelvis as you relax your pelvic floor. Imagine that you can breathe your baby out. You may also find this visualization very helpful in labor.

Benefits. The pelvic floor exercise involves both building strength and tone in the pelvic floor muscles, by contracting them, and learning to relax these muscles at will ("letting go"). Maintaining good tone of the pelvic floor is essential for a woman's health and well-being, especially during pregnancy, when the pelvic floor muscles support all the contents of the pelvis and abdomen. Problems caused by weakness of the pelvic floor, such as prolapse of the uterus, bowel, or bladder, can be prevented or reduced by this exercise, and varicosities can be relieved. The exercise also improves the blood circulation, to this area and reduces the risk of perineal tearing or injury during the birth. Knowing how to relax your pelvic floor muscles is very helpful when your baby is being born and the head needs to pass through these muscles. Practiced daily during pregnancy, the pelvic floor exercise greatly reduces the risk of damage to the pelvic floor during birth and promotes rapid recovery postnatally. Resume daily practice as soon as possible after the birth, and continue for a few weeks thereafter. The pelvic floor exercise should be practiced regularly throughout a woman's life.

Exercise Sequence VIII: Spinal Release

(Caution: This exercise sequence can be practiced up until six weeks before your due date, when you should stop lying on your back to exercise [see page 63].).

A. Basic Reclining Position

1. Lie on your back with your knees bent and your feet 12 inches apart, with your heels close to your buttocks. Turn out your heels slightly so the outsides of your feet are parallel. Place your hands on your lower belly. Relax your eyes, jaw, shoulders, and the back of your neck, bringing your chin down towards your chest.

2. Breathe deeply, dropping the back of your waist down onto the floor. Feel the soft downwards movement of your belly as you exhale, then its gentle expansion towards your hands as you inhale. Continue breathing deeply for a few moments, letting go of tension until you are deeply relaxed.

B. Pelvic Lift

1. Lie in the basic reclining position, and place your arms by your sides with the palms down. Drop your heels down onto the floor.

2. Keeping your feet firm and parallel, lift up your pelvis towards the ceiling as you exhale, lengthening your sacrum and lifting your spine

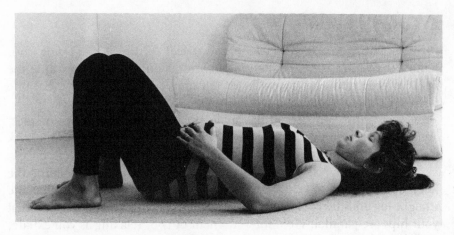

Exercise VIII A: Basic reclining position

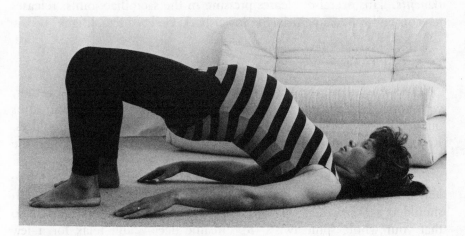

Exercise VIII B: Pelvic lift

until your weight is softly resting on your neck and shoulders and your feet. Keep your neck and shoulders completely relaxed. Breathe in slowly.

3. Now exhale, and slowly uncurl your spine, releasing one vertebra at a time from the neck downwards until all of your spine is in contact with the floor once more. Take a relaxing breath.

4. Repeat three times.

C. Lower Back Release

1. As you lie on your back, lift your feet off the floor. Using your hands, draw your knees gently towards your shoulders without lifting the back of your pelvis off the floor or tensing your shoulders (a). Breathe deeply for a few moments, releasing tension in your lower back.

2. Now cross your feet at the ankles, place your hands by your sides, and roll your hips, making a few circles on the floor with your lower back (b). Come back to the center, and repeat in the opposite direction.

3. Extend your left leg onto the floor, and bend the right, holding the knee and drawing it gently towards your shoulder (c). Ensure that the straight leg and the back of the pelvis remain down on the floor, and that your hips are parallel. Hold for a moment or two, relaxing as you exhale, and then change legs.

Benefits. This exercise releases pressure in the sacroiliac joints, releases tension and relieves pain in the lower back, and reduces fatigue.

D. Spinal Twist

1. As you lie on your back, raise both knees. Bring your feet together, with your heels as close to your buttocks as possible. Spread your arms out to the sides, palms down, so your arms are in line with your shoulders. Relax your shoulders and spine down onto the floor, and lengthen the back of your neck by tucking in your chin (a).

2. Breathe deeply, and, on an exhalation, turn your lower body to the left, bringing your knees down to the floor, while your arms and both shoulders stay in contact with the floor. Turn your head to the right so that your whole spine twists (b). Breathe deeply and relax for a few moments.

3. Come back to the center. Take a few deep breaths, relaxing your spine towards the floor with each exhalation.

4. Turn the other way—knees to the right and head to the left.

5. Come back to the center.

With a partner. Your partner can assist you with this exercise by sitting on your right side to begin with, and holding your right shoulder down with her left hand before you turn. Then, once you have rolled your lower body over to the left, she can place her right hand on your hip

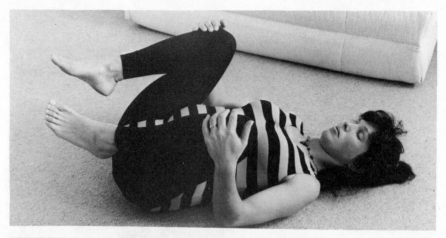

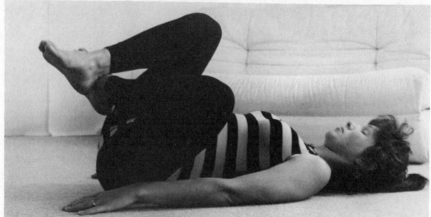

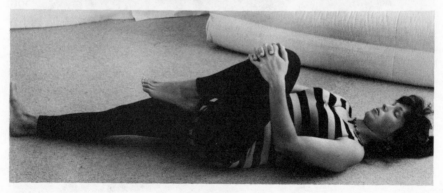

Exercise VIII C: Lower back release (a, b, *and* c)

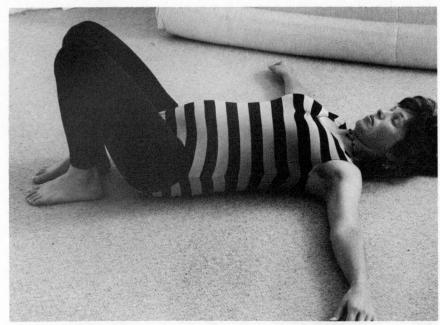

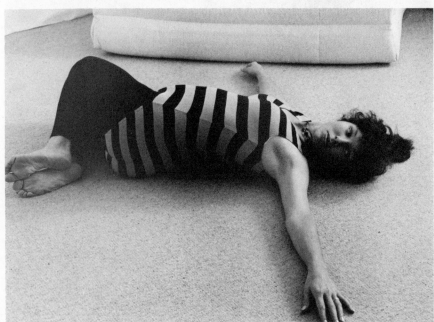

Exercise VIII D: Spinal twist

bone and gently, without pushing, assist you to rotate your legs downwards while keeping your shoulders in contact with the floor. Let go of tension as you breathe deeply.

Hold for a few moments, and then repeat on the other side, with your partner on your left.

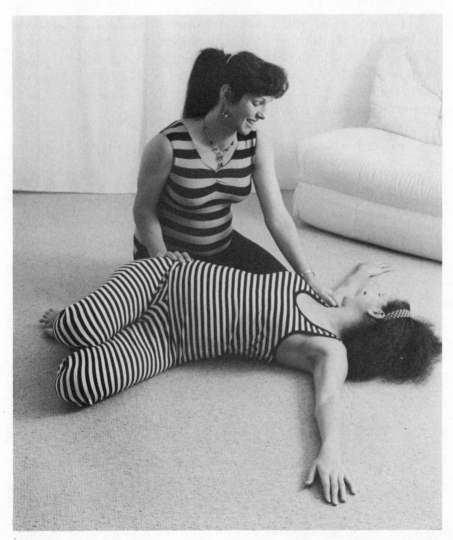

Spinal twist with partner

Benefits. The spinal twist gently turns the whole spinal column, stretching and releasing the muscles and intervertebral joints. This strengthens the spine and relieves tension in the lower back. When practiced regularly, the exercise reduces stiffness throughout the spine, from the neck to the tailbone.

E. Relaxation

1. Lie on your side with a cushion under your head and another under the bent knee of your top leg so that you are completely comfortable. Close your eyes, and allow all your body weight to drop comfortably onto the floor. Breathe deeply, relaxing each part of your body in turn with each exhalation. Keeping your awareness focused on your breathing, find your center as you relax more and more deeply.

Remain this way for 5 to 20 minutes.

2. Before you come up, focus your awareness on your baby inside you, and spend a few minutes in peaceful relaxation together.

3. When you are finished, take your time to open your eyes, letting the light come in slowly instead of hurrying to look outwards. Keep the sense of inner peace and relaxation as you stretch out slowly and come up in your own time.

Follow your exercise session with a drink of fruit juice, mineral water, or herbal tea. Avoid rushing about immediately after exercising. Ideally, follow the session with a swim, a bath, or a walk in the open air.

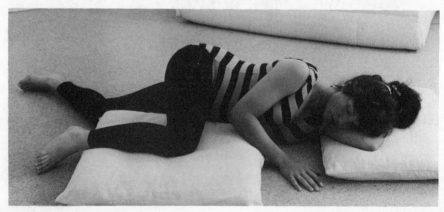

Exercise VIII E: Relaxation

4 | Breathing

THIS BOOK DOES NOT INCLUDE ANY SPECIAL BREATHING techniques for labor and birth. Instead, my aim is to ensure that you are breathing healthily (see exercise sequence I, page 47). In the same way that stiffness is an epidemic in our culture, restricted breathing is another!

With our modern way of living, our daily lives rarely demand that we use our bodies to their full capacities. Many of us spend our days without physically exerting ourselves enough to stimulate healthy breathing. The result is that our breathing may become shallower and faster than it should normally be, our supply of oxygen may be limited, and our elimination of carbon dioxide may be impaired.

If you observe the natural breathing of a baby or a young child, you will soon see that the abdomen is moving like a bellows with each breath, while the chest is relatively still and the shoulders are relaxed. This is natural, relaxed, deep breathing. By the time we reach adulthood many of us breathe too shallowly, using mainly the upper part of the chest rather than the abdomen, and approximately a third of our capacity for air. By breathing more rapidly than we should, we are taking in a new breath before we have emptied our lungs of stale air, so that some stale air is mixed with the fresh air we breathe in. This decreases our supply of oxygen. It also decreases our vitality.

We depend upon our breathing for life and health itself—breathing is a basic rhythm of our bodies. Each time we inhale, we are drawing in air—the life-giving element; each time we exhale, we are ridding ourselves of waste. This constant give and take, this flow of energy, starts the moment we are born and continues throughout our lives, pulsating within us like an alternating current. Every other activity of the body is closely connected with our breathing.

WHAT HAPPENS WHEN WE BREATHE?

The gateway to the air passages is the nose. Tiny hairs in the nostrils prevent dust particles from entering the lungs. The nasal passage, lined with mucous membranes, warm the air and filter out dust and germs. Glands fight off the bacteria, while our sense of smell protects us from inhaling harmful gases.

The muscles directly involved in breathing are the diaphragm, the strong partition of muscle separating the chest and the abdomen, and the intercostal muscles, between the ribs. The lungs themselves contain no muscles; they expand into the empty space around them, the thoracic cavity. The strong membrane that envelops the lungs connects them with the walls of the chest, whose movements cause the lungs to expand and contract as air is inhaled and exhaled.

When we breath shallowly, we are mainly using the intercostal muscles. When we breathe deeply, the diaphragm muscle moves rhythmically up and down as well, allowing the thoracic cavity to expand fully.

Efficient breathing depends on good posture. If your chest is constricted and your shoulders hunched, the space in your thoracic cavity is less and your breathing is impaired.

Shaped like a vault, the diaphragm muscle flattens out when it works, pressing the abdominal organs downward and the abdomen outwards as you breathe in. When you exhale it relaxes, arching upwards towards the chest cavity. This is what you feel as you breathe deeply, your belly expanding with the in-breath and retracting with the out-breath. By moving up and down with each breath, the diaphragm puts mild pressure on the liver, the stomach, and other internal organs. The rhythm of the lungs is transformed into a gentle massage that promotes the natural

Inhalation (left): as air enters the lungs, the diaphragm moves down and pressure in the abdomen increases.

Exhalation (right): as air leaves the lungs, the diaphragm moves up and pressure in the abdomen decreases.

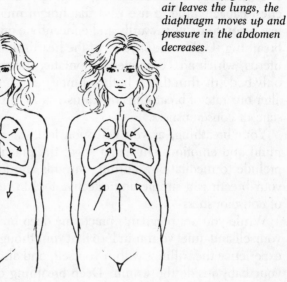

functioning of the internal organs. Every breath stimulates the blood circulation to these organs and improves the metabolism. This beneficial massage is lacking when we breathe merely with our upper chest.

Although we can survive for weeks without solid foods and several days without water, life without air is only possible for a few minutes. Every living cell absorbs oxygen and expels it in the form of carbon dioxide. In pregnancy and labor you are breathing for your body and also for your baby.

BREATHING DURING LABOR

Normally we breathe in and out through the nose. In the deep breathing exercise (chapter 3, exercise sequence I), I recommend exhaling through the mouth. This is because during strong contractions in labor, as in all vigorous activity, most women naturally tend to breathe out through their mouths. So while you usually breathe in and out through your nose without thinking about it, you might like to breathe out through your mouth when you practice the deep breathing exercise, or if you feel like it in labor or occasionally while exercising. Regular practice of this exercise will deepen your breathing, helping you to breathe with your whole chest capacity and to use your diaphragm muscle correctly. It will also teach you to focus inwardly and concentrate on the basic rhythm of your breathing. Unlike the rhythm of the heartbeat, or the contractions of the uterus, which are completely automatic, the rhythm of the breath is the only body rhythm that is both voluntary and involuntary. We are able to alter our rate of breathing consciously, and this has a direct effect on our state of consciousness.

Your breathing, as you will soon feel, is very closely linked to your mind and emotions. In hatha yoga, the practice of deep breathing is a prelude to meditation. Turning inwards and focusing your attention on your breath is a simple and effective tool for experiencing deeper states of consciousness.

While you are pregnant, practicing deep breathing helps you to calm yourself and quiet your mind, so that your thoughts subside. You can then experience the stillness within yourself, and also focus on the presence of your baby inside the womb. Deep breathing can deepen your sense of the peaceful and pleasurable times of the pregnancy and help when you feel anxious or out of sorts.

In labor, breathing can help you to cope with the deep and intense feelings you experience. There are no special techniques you need to remember for labor; your breathing can be spontaneous. However, if during labor you feel tense, anxious, or fearful, you can use deep breathing to calm and center yourself and to focus your awareness inwards. This will help you to ignore what is going on around you and to achieve the state of consciousness that is appropriate to labor.

Focusing on breathing deeply is also a powerful help when the contractions begin to get painful. By concentrating on long, slow exhalations through the peaks of the contractions, you will find it easier to stay relaxed during contractions and also to rest in between them. As contractions increase in intensity, you may find it helpful to release low, deep sounds along with the exhalations, besides using the movements and positions suggested in chapter 6. Breathing this way will help you to express the pain rather than keeping it all inside and becoming tense and overwhelmed.

Many mothers tell me that concentrating on breathing has helped them to cope with their labors. In the words of one mother, "Through each contraction I used the deep breathing, at times quite fast and noisily but always with concentration and awareness of the peak and then the fading of the pain. I was very aware of exactly where the baby was and how my body was doing, and people remarked afterwards how relaxed all my body had been apart from the contracting muscles."

Practicing deep breathing regularly in pregnancy will enhance your ability to focus on your breathing rhythm in labor. The more you practice ahead of time, the easier it will become to use your breathing without any special mental effort on the day. Like meditation techniques, deep breathing becomes a more powerful tool with regular practice. And it is wonderful to practice your breathing with the partner who will be with you when you give birth.

When you begin to practice deep breathing, at first you will enjoy a pleasant feeling of calm and relaxation. After a time this feeling will deepen into a blissful meditation, uniting your mind and body and enhancing your awareness of your child within. This is very much like the peace between contractions during labor. Deep breathing will also help you to relax when you are learning to feed and care for your baby in the days and weeks after the birth.

5 | Massage

COMBINED WITH MOVEMENT, POSITIONS, AND BREATH-ing, massage can be of great use to you in pregnancy and labor. For many people there is nothing as comforting and soothing as the touch of another. Your hands can surprise you with the relaxing, healing power they contain. By touching we can express our love and affection for each other, and we can also relieve ourselves and others of aches and pains and unnecessary muscle tension.

Massage is an art that needs to be cultivated, and the only way to learn is through exploration and experiment. There are many different kinds of massage, but in this book we will explore the simplest, "intuitive" massage, without using any specific methods.

Start on your own body. Discover what feels good and which parts of your body need massage, and then work with another, preferably someone who will be with you during labor. Always bear in mind that whereas some women love being massaged in labor and find it a helpful way of relieving pain, others prefer not to be touched. It is impossible to know in advance when, how, or even if you will want to be touched in labor. Sometimes massage in labor can be distracting or annoying, but many women do find it very comforting and very helpful as a form of pain relief. You will probably enjoy practicing massage during pregnancy, and you can decide at the time what is most appropriate for labor.

There are four basic kinds of massage:

Surface stroking. This is usually done with the flat of the hand. In severe pain or spasm or on a young baby or child, this very light stroking is often the only form of massage possible.

Deep stroking. This is done in the same way as surface stroking, but more firmly, using greater pressure.

Deep pressure. This is done by pressing firmly with the tips of your fingers or thumbs, or even your knuckles or elbows, over a small area at a time, reaching deep to tense spots in the body and, sometimes, using small circular movements to loosen them. Deep massage works on muscle tissue and bone rather than the skin.

Kneading. This is done by using your whole hand to alternately squeeze and release a muscle. It is useful over large muscle areas such as buttocks or thighs.

A good place to start is with your own hands and feet:

Hand Massage

1. Using one hand, explore the skin surface of the other and the bony structure underneath. Explore the range of movement of all the joints. Bend each finger backwards and forwards, and gently pull and twist it. Then separate your fingers from side to side.

2. Now explore deeply into the spaces between the bones of the back of your hand and your wrist bones.

3. Last, shake your hands rapidly, allowing the movement to start from your shoulders. Keep your whole arm relaxed, your wrists completely loose.

4. Massage your other hand the same way.

Now explore your feet in the same way.

Foot Massage

1. Using your thumbs, try different degrees of pressure. Press all the way up the arch of your instep as firmly as you can, making small circular movements with your thumb. If you find a painful spot, work on it for a while and try to dissolve the painful sensations. You will probably feel little crystal-like knots under the skin that yield to the firm massage and seem to disappear.

2. Try the same thing all around the base of your big toe, the sole of your foot, and then your ankle and calf.

3. Finally, explore the top of your foot and then your toes, one by one, bending them first backwards and then forwards, extending each joint to its limit. Then pull them and twist them, and finally separate them from side to side.

4. Massage the other foot the same way.

Once you have enjoyed massaging your own feet, treat your partner to a foot massage. The two of you may then enjoy experimenting with different parts of the body, neck and shoulders, back and front. You will find that with experience, your enjoyment will grow, as your own natural inventiveness leads the way. As your interest grows you may want to consult one of the many good books on massage (see "Recommended Reading"). Courses in massage are also widely available.

MASSAGE FOR PREGNANCY

Massage is particularly beneficial during pregnancy, when the added weight of your belly and the increase in body fluids can result in stress and discomfort. The lower back, the shoulders, and the feet are especially vulnerable. Regular massage makes it much easier to adapt to the enormous changes your body undergoes in these months.

Self-Massage

After your bath explore your whole body, perhaps oiling your skin, particularly your belly and breasts, with a good vegetable oil such as almond or wheat-germ. This, along with exercise and good nutrition, will make stretch marks less likely.

In the last month of pregnancy some midwives recommend oiling and gently stretching the perineum each day after a bath in preparation for birth. It will be helpful to be familiar with your pelvic area, to explore the bones of your pelvis and massage away any tension in your groin. You may want to feel your cervix (try this gently after bathing, in the squatting position).

While you exercise, gently massage the part of your body where you are feeling the stretch. This is particularly useful for the inner thighs.

With a Partner

Practicing massage with a partner is especially beneficial before sleep. It is also perfect preparation for massaging your baby after birth.

To warm up, try this:

Head and Neck Massage

(Caution: Although lying on your back may be comfortable in early pregnancy, you should avoid the reclining position in late pregnancy, in labor, and at any time it makes you feel dizzy or uncomfortable. During these times, your partner can massage your neck and shoulders while you are sitting upright or kneeling.)

Lie on your back on the floor with your knees bent and legs up on a chair or bed. Place your arms down comfortably by your sides. Have your partner sit or kneel behind you; make sure that he or she too is comfortable. (Alternatively, you can lie on a bed while your partner sits on a chair behind you.) Your partner should follow these instructions:

1. With your hands, press downwards on her shoulders to help her relax them as she breathes out. Now slip your hands behind her neck, and stroke firmly upwards from the base of the neck towards the head, alternating hands. Repeat a few times, lengthening the neck.

2. Go back over the same area, but this time make small circles with your fingertips, working your way slowly up the neck.

3. Then lift up her head in your hands and press it slowly and gently upwards and forwards so that her chin comes down towards her breast-

bone. Hold for a second or two, and then slowly lower her head to the floor. Now turn the head gently to one side, and stroke firmly up the side of the neck, ending up with firm circular movements at the base of the skull. Linger there for a while, then turn the head to the other side, and repeat.

4. Now explore the jaw bone, the upper jaw and mouth, cheeks, cheekbones, nose, temples, and the rims of the eye sockets. In each area, make even stroking movements from the center outwards. Then go over the same area, making firmer, small, circular movements and exerting more pressure.

5. Stroke the brow from the center outwards, and finally place your hands on either side of the head with your fingers gently covering the eyelids. Sit quietly like this for a minute, as both of you breathe deeply, and then gently, gently lift your hands.

Back Massage

This massage is blissful in late pregnancy and during labor. Because the nerves that run to the pelvis stem from the lower lumbar and sacral parts of the spine, massaging the lower back, especially, can be an effective way of relieving pain during contractions. You will probably want your partner to massage during contractions, and to stop in between. You may want deep pressure massage, or you may prefer a light stroking. You may want motionless pressure applied to your coccyx. You and your partner can practice all of these in the following exercise. For labor, have on hand a pleasant-smelling talcum powder, cornstarch, or massage oil to avoid stickiness.

To practice back massage, rest comfortably in the kneeling position, leaning forward onto a pile of cushions, with your knees apart and your feet pointing towards each other. Your partner should kneel behind you, keeping his or her own back straight. (Alternatively, sit facing backwards on a chair. Your partner can kneel behind you on the floor or sit on another chair.)

Have your partner follow these instructions:

1. Starting at the base of the skull, feel each vertebra of the spine, massaging each one in small circles. Work downwards until you reach the sacrum.

2. Using the thumbs of each hand, massage the muscles on the sides

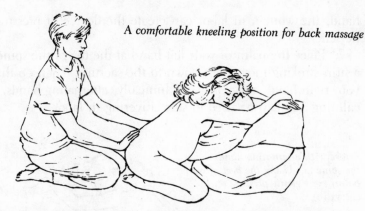

A comfortable kneeling position for back massage

of the spinal column, using as firm a pressure as your partner can enjoy, again making small circular movements. Linger on the tense spots.

3. Place your hands on the soft muscles in the shoulders, and knead until tension yields.

4. Using the flat surface of your palm, particularly the heel, make light, slow, rhythmic circles over the sacral area, increasing pressure according to your partner's needs. Try to harmonize your strokes with her breathing. The best way to practice this is to breathe deeply yourself while you massage.

5. Now, using the palms of both hands and starting at the center of her lower back, make slow, even movements outwards towards or even down her thighs. Then lift your hands, and repeat.

6. Cup one hand over the lower end of the spine so that the heel of your palm covers her coccyx. Keeping your hand still, exert slight pressure, so that the warmth of your hand spreads into her back. Some women find this helpful during contractions. By moving her body against her partner's

Use one hand to massage in a circular movement on the lower back (a). *Use both hands to stroke outwards from the sacrum, down the thighs and calves* (b).

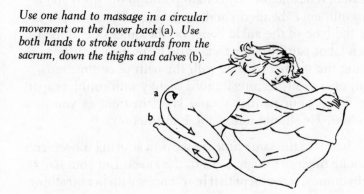

hand, the woman in labor can create the degree of pressure she needs herself.

7. Place the palm of your left hand at the top of the spine, and make a firm stroking movement down to the sacrum. Then do the same with your right hand, and repeat rhythmically, alternating hands. This is very calming and can be used to stop shivering in labor.

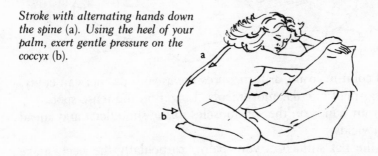

Stroke with alternating hands down the spine (a). *Using the heel of your palm, exert gentle pressure on the coccyx* (b).

Thigh, Calf, and Foot Massage

The muscles of the inner thigh often tense up in labor, and some women feel the pain of contractions in this area. Gentle stroking helps relax the adductors, or inner thigh muscles, assisting the opening of the cervix and the release of tension in the whole pelvic area.

Massaging the calves can prevent or reduce leg cramps during pregnancy and help to relieve tiredness and edema in the feet.

Foot massage is also very comforting in pregnancy, when the feet may ache from carrying extra weight. Massaging the feet may be very helpful during labor, as well; reflexologists say certain points in the heels and the Achilles' tendons influence the uterus and genital area. For some people, deep massage at the base of the ankle bone, on the outer side of the leg can help to lessen labor pain. Foot massage also helps the whole body to relax, thus helping the mother to cope with the pain of contractions.

Sit comfortably on a chair, leaning forward slightly with your legs apart and feet on the floor. Your partner should kneel in front of you in a comfortable position. He should follow these instructions:

1. Using both hands at the same time, make firm stroking movements from the groin along the inner thigh, towards the knees. Lift your hands, and repeat in a rhythmical movement that harmonizes with her breathing.

2. Now take one of her feet and place it in your lap. With one hand, bend her toes up towards her leg. With the other hand, take hold of the calf muscles and gently knead them.

3. Now pass on to the foot. Holding it in one hand, use the other hand to make smooth circles over both sides of the heel, then even strokes on either side of the achilles tendon, behind the ankle bone. Do this only very lightly in pregnancy, since deep massage of the heels can stimulate uterine contractions, according to some reflexologists. Deeper massage can safely be used in labor to enhance contractions and relieve pain.

4. Switch feet, and massage her other calf and foot.

Belly Massage

During labor, while you are experiencing the intense sensations of a contraction, you may find a light fingertip massage over your lower abdomen soothing. Try this yourself in the standing position.

Make a very gentle sweeping movement over your lower belly, in a half circle from one side to the other. Lift your hand, and repeat in harmony with your breathing.

Now have your partner try it.

Lastly, your partner should become familiar with the parts of your body that generally tense up when you are under stress, and be able intuitively to stroke away your tension in labor, be it a frown on your forehead, tense, raised shoulders, clenched fists, or whatever.

Many women enjoy the relaxing effect of massage in labor. However, you may find that you prefer not to be touched when the time comes, or that massage becomes too distracting. You might prefer a very light touch, or you might enjoy a deeper pressure. Make your likes and dislikes known to your partner, and don't be afraid to ask for what you want, as this is the only way he or she will know how best to help you.

6 | Labor and Birth

FOR THE SAKE OF CONVENIENCE, LABOR AND BIRTH CAN be described in three stages: the dilation of the cervix, or opening of the uterus, is referred to as the first stage of labor; the expulsive stage—when the child is born—is known as the second stage; and the first contact between you and your baby, followed by the expulsion of the placenta and membranes, is the third stage.

In the last few weeks before labor starts, you will begin to feel your uterus contracting. These prelabor, "practice" contractions (known as Braxton-Hicks contractions) are usually painless. As you feel your uterus tighten within, with your hands you can feel your abdomen harden on the outside. This tightening can last for fifteen minutes or longer and may be most noticeable after vigorous activity. However, not all women are aware of this increase in uterine activity in the last weeks of pregnancy.

At any time within the last six weeks of pregnancy, your baby's head will probably "engage" in the pelvic inlet, where it is ready for birth. You might feel some strong contractions when this happens. The baby's head may not engage until labor starts, particularly if this is a second or subsequent baby. Some women experience frequent mild contractions a day or so before going into labor; often continuing for a few hours and then ceasing, these are known as prelabor. It is important to expect the possibility of prelabor. If you are doubtful as to whether your contractions are the real thing, they probably are not!

The big question is: How will you know when labor is starting? Established labor starts when your cervix begins to dilate beyond 2 centimeters. The buildup to labor is usually slow and gradual. Here are some of the ways labor can begin:

1. It may start with a "show," which is a discharge of blood-stained mucus, the plug that sealed your cervical opening during pregnancy. This mucous plug can come away before labor starts or at any time during the first stage. If the plug comes away at the same time that the membranes break, the amniotic fluid may be a little blood-stained at first, but should soon become colorless.

2. Sometimes the first thing to happen is the breaking of the membranes, or leaking of the waters. It may come as a huge gush of amniotic fluid or a slow leaking of the water in front of the baby, known as the forewaters. This, too, may not happen until well on in the first stage, or it can happen 24 hours or more before labor actually begins. (If contractions haven't started after 12 hours, your risk of infection is increased. Vaginal exams should be avoided, and it is wise to keep very clean. Wash down after each visit to the toilet, and avoid lying in the bathtub; take a shower or kneel upright in the bath instead. Seven or eight garlic tablets and 1 gram of vitamin C, taken every two to three hours, will help prevent infection.) Sometimes the membranes remain intact until the moment of birth—or even afterward, so the baby is born in a caul. Most commonly, membranes break just before the second stage.

"I felt a 'pop,' and warm waters flooded out of me. I felt instantly wide awake and excited."

3. Labor may start as persistent, dull backache caused by the contractions of the uterus.

4. The first sign of labor may be diarrhea, as the bowels have a natural tendency to empty before labor starts.

5. Labor may begin with shivering and shakiness. This is the body's way of letting out tension. It often happens at the start of labor, though it may occur at any point during labor. The best thing to do is just let it pass, breathing deeply and perhaps having your back or feet massaged.

6. The most reliable sign that labor has started is contractions. These

will be somewhat stronger than the prelabor contractions. They might feel similar to menstrual pains, in the lower abdomen, or else you may feel them in your lower back or inner thighs.

> *"I became slowly aware of that familiar tightening and mild cramp in my abdomen. I had been in a sound sleep until this point, so I didn't immediately realize things had begun. But as I continued to experience these pains at five-minute intervals, more or less, it was soon obvious that the baby was on the way."*

The first contractions may feel quite uncomfortable, or they may be so mild that you can sleep through them or remain unaware of them. Contractions are experienced very differently by different women, and even by the same woman in different labors. They may be mild or strong when they start. They may come every half hour or every 10 minutes, or perhaps at quite irregular intervals. Your uterus will begin to contract and tighten; the cervix will thin and draw up, and then slowly open. Some women describe contractions as "rushes of energy." Each one comes on like a wave—starting out, building up to a peak, and tailing off. At its peak the contraction can be painful, but there will be a rest before the next one starts. It helps to think of waves on the shore.

> *"The contractions were still very mild and ten minutes apart when I arrived at the hospital. The nursing staff were reluctant to admit me, as they said I appeared to be so calm they weren't even sure I was in labor.*
>
> *"I walked about and squatted, and when I was next examined thirty minutes later they seemed to be amazed that I was progressing so quickly. The contractions were now five minutes apart and quite strong, and I found that by leaning forward against the wall and also kneeling on all fours on the floor I got a lot of relief."*

As the labor progresses, the contractions become more frequent and more intense, with shorter gaps between them. By the time you are in well-established labor, the contractions will be really intense and you will need to give them all your attention.

> *"The contractions became a lot more demanding of me. I mostly sat upright on the edge of my bed, leaning forward on a chair back, as I concentrated on deep belly breathing."*

"I started getting pains, rather like bad menstrual pains, every ten minutes. I found that by breathing deeply through them I could easily cope with them. Between the pains I kept myself active at first, doing things around the house, but as the contractions got stronger I needed to rest over a pile of cushions in the gaps between."

THE SENSATIONS OF LABOR

Birth is a very special event in your sexual life as a woman. It is a time when you are transformed: you become a mother; you give birth to another human being. As your womb opens up completely during labor, you will also experience a change in your normal consciousness. In the hours of labor you may have trouble focusing on day-to-day affairs; your attention will naturally turn inwards, as if the whole world contracts to what is happening within your body. In your mind, time takes on a fresh dimension. Hours can pass in what seems like minutes; you may feel "outside of time," as one woman described it. It is like being in another world.

This great opening of the womb happens only once or a few times in your life. It is a very deep emotional experience that involves a regression to your most basic feelings, as if everything you have ever been through is part of the present time. There is, perhaps, an unconscious remembrance of once being in the womb yourself, of being born, and of being a very small child. Yet at the same time you feel the dawning of yourself as a mother, and a very intimate communion between you and your body and your child within. Your womb is the seat of your deepest feelings. In the same way that you need to sink deeply into your inner feelings when you experience full sexual orgasm, you need to respond instinctively to the urges and messages of your body when you are in labor and about to give birth.

In a way, you need to lose control, to surrender to and trust in the birth process, which takes place without your conscious control. You need to let go of your mind, of everything that you know, and just let it happen. This is a time to turn inwards, to abandon oneself to the un-known, not to think ahead of what is to come. Take it moment by moment, and let the natural, involuntary rhythms of your body take over. As one mother said, "if you relax, you float, if you struggle and fight, you sink."

You will probably experience intense feelings of every kind, from agony to ecstasy, from despair and weakness to courage and strength, from exhaustion to incredible energy and power. You are also likely to experience some nausea. Although some women never do, others experience a lot during labor. This is nothing to be afraid of; in fact, retching and vomiting can be a great relief, and can help free you of tension and anxiety. Birth is a great emptying, so it should not be surprising that your stomach and bowels tend to empty themselves of their contents at this time. In fact, vomiting can be a sign of fast dilation. You will also need to empty your bladder every hour or so in labor, as a full bladder can get in the baby's way as the head descends into the pelvic cavity.

LIFE-GIVING PAIN

The pain of childbirth has a bad reputation. There is no doubt about it: as any experienced mother will tell you, giving birth is usually painful. It is certainly realistic to expect pain, even though you may turn out to be one of the lucky few who doesn't feel any—and there are some! Most women experience pain at the peak of contractions. The pains are acute rather than throbbing and continuous, and do not generally last in between contractions. Often a very strong contraction is followed by a milder one. The pain is not the same as that of injury. Many women describe the pain as "positive" or "life-giving," with pleasure to equal it between contractions.

One of the main causes of unnecessary pain in childbirth is the use of the reclining position. Even if you are propped up by pillows, when you are reclining you are like a stranded beetle—completely helpless—and the contractions of your uterus hurt more. Other postures, such as kneeling forward, standing, squatting, or sitting upright, actually relieve the pain and help you tune in to what is happening inside you. You need the freedom to use your whole body to discover how to make yourself comfortable.

> "I felt incredibly uncomfortable whenever I lay down, and being in an upright position was the only way I could fully concentrate on trying to relax and keep up the deep breathing."

> "I found small movements helpful—at one point I found I was almost dancing. Leaning against anything hard was impossible for me, and lying on my back was the worst thing of all."

Often it is the wrong kind of environment and atmosphere that causes extra pain. During pregnancy and labor your body produces hormones called endorphins, which are natural relaxants and pain relievers. Another hormone secreted by your body is oxytocin, which stimulates the contractions and the birth process. However, the secretion of these hormones is deeply connected with your emotions. Your body will produce more of these hormones if you feel secure, relaxed, uninhibited, and free to be yourself. A feeling of being watched can inhibit hormonal secretions and make you tense up as well. These are vital considerations when choosing the attendants and place of birth. The presence of unnecessary people in the room, or someone you do not feel relaxed with, can interfere with the labor process. For some women total privacy is essential.

> *"The positions had left me feeling very uninhibited, and because I was at home I felt very safe and comfortable. I moaned and groaned and released the power that way, too—it felt wonderful. I was an intuitive instrument for the birth—Toby was coming, and my body just opened up."*

It is important for you to have help from people you trust. You need the comfort and support of your husband or someone close to you in labor. Even women with an intense need to be alone in labor want attendants or a partner nearby in case they are needed. Others need the supporting partner close at hand.

> *"With constant encouragement from my husband and the midwife, I felt spurred on to my goal. Ismail said afterwards that he was glad that he could help me—such as by bringing me back to my deep breathing whenever I lost control of it."*

I have already discussed the change of consciousness that happens in the first stage of labor. It is very helpful to be in semidarkness at this time, with a minimum of unnecessary sensory stimulation. Soft, soothing music may help you, and your attendants as well. Immersing yourself in water is one of the most effective ways of relieving pain in labor. The use of a pool is ideal; otherwise have a bathtub or shower available. If you feel stuck or inhibited, then try taking a warm bath (see chapter 8).

> *"The bath was a big help, and I found myself rotating my hips and massaging my tummy. I had a mental picture then of stroking and comforting the baby inside me through its ordeal. We were both, after all, in the same boat!"*

There is a definite correlation between anxiety and fear, on the one hand, and pain, on the other. When you are afraid or cold or overexcited, your body secretes adrenaline, a hormone that inhibits the birth process during labor (although it may play a helpful part during the onset of the second stage). Your muscles tense up, your breathing becomes shallow; you are trying to run away from what is happening inside you. This increases the pain. As soon as you relax and go with it, the pain lessens.

Good preparation of body and mind during pregnancy helps you to approach birth with confidence. Practicing the yoga-based exercises during pregnancy ensures that you are physically fit for birth and enables you to make friends with your pain and to release some of it before the day of the birth. Focusing your awareness on your breathing and your inner self will teach you to still your mind and to surrender to the powerful sensations inside you.

No two labors are alike: the size and shape of your baby and the position in which he or she is lying will make a difference in the pain you feel (see page 184). Labor pain is a very subjective experience as well; we all have differing abilities to tolerate it. Some women will talk of unexpected depths of pain during labor, while others will say they couldn't really call it pain at all.

> *"The pain was worse than I had imagined—it was much fiercer. I felt I was being taken up by a giant hand and shaken over a raging black sea. But just when I thought I was going to drown I would be pulled back by the eyes of my friend, who had been through the experience already and knew something of what I was going through."*

> *"I found the birth a marvelous experience—not at all painful, only uncomfortable. It was marvelous being able to move about and remain upright. I felt in control most of the time."*

When birth is active, when the environment is conducive, and when the attendants are sensitive and considerate, the pain is certainly much more tolerable. In these ideal circumstances very few women need or ask for pain-relieving drugs, even when these are easily available.

It is always wise, though, when approaching such an unknown adventure, to keep an open mind. If you find the pain intolerable, the birth may be a more positive experience if you accept the help of pain-relieving drugs. These do, however, enter the bloodstream of your baby and have certain side effects, which you need to consider carefully (see page 196). Some of the effects on your baby can be harmful, so do find out as much as you can about the drugs available—their pros and cons and how to make the best use of them. There are helpful homeopathic remedies that do not have harmful effects (see page 197).

Time and again I have heard mothers say, "Even though it was painful, it was worth it!"

"This birth I found so different from that of my first baby. Then I had been encouraged to have Demerol, and I found that this made me very sleepy—not at all in control. This time, having had no drugs, I remained alert and felt very much in touch with my body, although I do think that the pain was more acute."

Occasionally women say that the moment of birth was like the greatest orgasm they have ever experienced. Women talk of great ecstasy and bliss, of the deepest feelings of joy and love.

"A sense of completion, relief, gratefulness, and joy filled me. Similar feelings were shared by my husband, and tears were running down his face."

It is important to realize that the pain involved is only part of the great variety of intense feelings one experiences. And if one cuts out the pain, one generally cuts out, to some extent, the other feelings too.

The greatest advantage of accepting and tolerating the pain, and allowing nature to take its course without disturbing the whole process, is the alert, healthy, undamaged, and vigorous baby you have at the end, and the good beginning to the relationship between you.

THE FIRST STAGE OF LABOR

Before labor begins, your baby lies within the uterus with his or her head resting in the pelvic brim, ready to be born. The cervix, or mouth of the uterus, is tightly closed, and sealed by a mucous plug. The membranes surrounding your baby are intact; they contain the fluid in which the baby floats. Before labor starts, the cervix is about 1½ inches thick. In the week or so before the birth, hormones secreted by your body will cause the cervix to soften and become "ripe," ready to open up in labor.

What Happens to Your Baby

Before the onset of labor your baby's head will probably engage in the pelvic brim. The widest diameter of the top of his or her head, from the crown to the forehead, will be lying in the widest diameter of your pelvic inlet, which is from side to side. As your cervix dilates, the baby's head gradually descends further into the pelvic cavity.

As it descends, your baby's head exerts pressure on the cervix; this pressure assists and promotes dilation. The dilating uterus pulls up around the baby's head like a glove as the baby goes down into the pelvic canal. By the time you are fully dilated, it will have drawn up around the baby's head as far as the ears and opened wide enough for the baby's body to pass through.

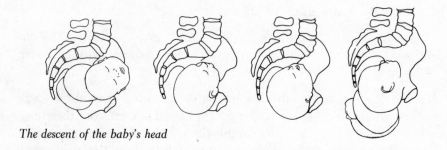

The descent of the baby's head

What Happens to You

When labor starts, the early contractions will draw up the cervix so that it thins out and becomes ready to open. Sometimes this thinning takes place in the days before labor actually begins—particularly with second and subsequent babies. You may have prelabor in the 24 hours or so preceding the birth, with mild contractions that stop and start periodically. Eventually the contractions will begin to take on a regular rhythm.

The "classic" labor starts with regular contractions, 20 to 30 minutes apart and 20 to 30 seconds long. After some time, as your cervix dilates, they progress to 15 minutes apart (30 to 35 seconds long), then 10 minutes apart (35 to 40 seconds long), 5 minutes apart (40 to 45 seconds long), 3 minutes apart (45 to 50 seconds long), until finally, at the end of the first

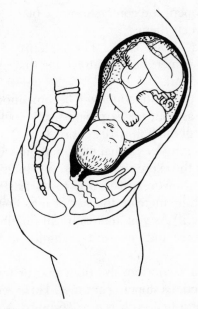

Before labor begins: the baby in the womb at term.

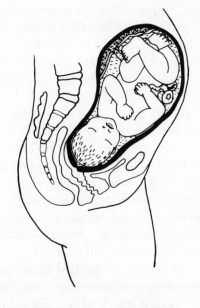

Labor begins: the cervix effaces and becomes thinner as early contractions draw it upwards.

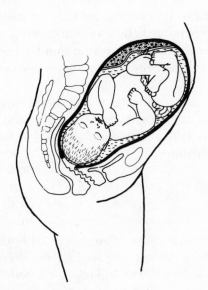

Early first stage: the cervix opens.

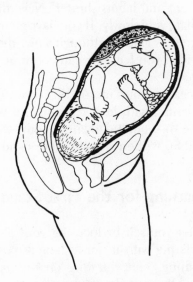

Late first stage: the cervix draws up around the baby's head.

stage, when the cervix is almost fully open, the contractions are 60 to 90 seconds long with half a minute between them.

However, very few women have a classic labor. The patterns and rhythms of labor vary greatly. Some women have contractions that are 10 minutes or 5 minutes apart throughout.

Whatever the rhythm of your labor, the contractions will become more powerful, longer, and closer together as your cervix progressively opens and dilates from 0 to 10 centimeters (full dilation is 10 centimeters). You or your midwife can feel the cervix dilating by vaginal examination with the hand, which is why you often hear the expression "four or five fingers dilated." (If labor is progressing well, however, it is wise to do as few internal examinations as possible, as they increase the risk of infection. Sometimes they are not necessary at all!) As you approach full dilation the contractions are at their most intense and you are nearing the time when your baby will be born.

The length of the first stage can vary enormously, from one or two hours to two or three days with contractions stopping at times. However, the average length of the first stage for a first birth is 8 to 16 hours.

Modern hospitals are reluctant to allow a labor to take longer than 24 hours and often use a Pitocin drip to accelerate a long labor. One of the benefits of active birth is that contractions tend to be more regular and efficient and labors shorter. Nevertheless, it is normal for some women to dilate very slowly. If you have plenty of rest in between contractions and progress is gradual, though slow, there should be no reason to intervene provided you feel you can continue and the baby is showing no signs of distress.

Because your uterus tilts forward as it contracts, it will work most efficiently, with least resistance, if you are upright and leaning forward. Being in a quiet darkened room, with as few people and distractions as possible, will encourage more rapid dilation.

Breathing for the First Stage

Center yourself by focusing your awareness on your breathing, without interfering with it, for as long as possible. When you need to, use deep breathing, concentrating on the exhalations. Try to keep your body, especially your shoulders, relaxed.

When the contractions become very intense you may need to make a

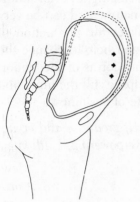

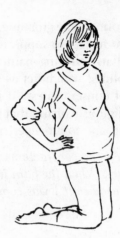

The uterus tilts forward as it contracts, so in an upright position there is no resistance to gravity.

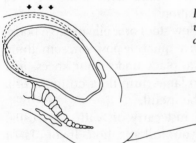

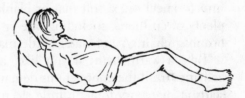

In the semireclining position, the uterus works against the pull of gravity as it contracts.

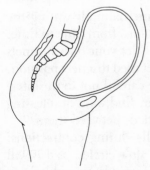

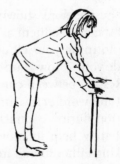

By standing (or kneeling) and leaning forward, you help the uterus to do its work with least resistance.

lot of sound, like groaning, moaning, humming, singing, or even shouting. Do not try to suppress this, as it is perfectly natural and can be very helpful in relieving pain. Making sound stimulates the production of endorphins, which act as natural pain relievers and help to change the level of consciousness. It is well known in various forms of meditation and religious worship that singing or chanting helps to still the mind and to bring one to a deeper, more concentrated state of awareness.

> *"As the contractions increased I found myself groaning and crying out. When the pain increased and became overpowering, I still knew inside that I was coping well."*

Positions and Movements for the First Stage of Labor

In early labor it is a good idea to loosen up by doing some of the exercises in this book. Leave out the reclining positions.

Arrange your room so that you have a low stool or a pile of large books to place under your buttocks for support in a squatting position, something firm to kneel on, a soft mat or blanket to place under your knees, and plenty of cushions, including one or two large, firm floor cushions or a beanbag chair. A hot water bottle may be useful.

Take a warm bath, if you like, and just carry on with your usual activities until the contractions demand your full attention. If your labor starts at night, try to get a little sleep. It will help you to conserve your energy for the really strong contractions to come. If you cannot sleep, then rest in a comfortable upright position on your bed, supported by pillows.

The positions shown in this section often come naturally during the first stage. Use them as a guide, and change positions from time to time. Try to make yourself comfortable and, above all, let your own instincts guide you. Allow yourself a few contractions to get used to a new position.

Resting between contractions is important! Be careful not to misinterpret the word *active* and exhaust yourself. Rather, find ways of releasing tension during contractions, and resting, supported, between them.

It may help to move your pelvis rhythmically during contractions, rocking either to and fro, from side to side, or in slow circles, as this will aid the dilation of your cervix and the descent of your baby and help to dissipate the pain.

"I felt the contractions so strongly that I could really only do one thing: walk, walk, walk—at quite a pace!"

Walking or Standing

Ambulation, or walking, shortens labor and increases the efficiency of contractions.[1] In the early part of the first stage, try to walk about, leaning forward for contractions.

"For the first stage I began by keeping upright and walking around the delivery room. During the contractions I leaned slightly forward and held onto the end of the bed while my husband massaged my back. I moved my hips in circles during the contractions. I didn't find them at all painful, only uncomfortable."

With your body vertical, the descent of the baby is helped by the downward force of gravity. Some women like to stand throughout labor—even for delivery. Others have remarked that holding onto a rope or pole and hanging minimizes the pain (there are records of women in non-Western societies doing the same thing). It can be helpful to put your arms around the shoulders of another person and hang. The sup-

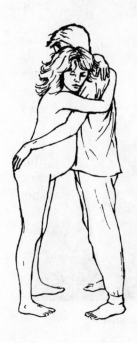

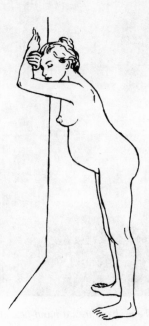

Your partner can hold you in the standing position, providing reassuring bodily contact as well as physical support, or you can lean against a wall.

porter should keep his or her shoulders relaxed, bend the knees slightly, and lean back while tucking the pelvis under to carry your weight without getting an aching back (see page 142). It is helpful to practice this beforehand. Many women find it comforting to be held as they stand during

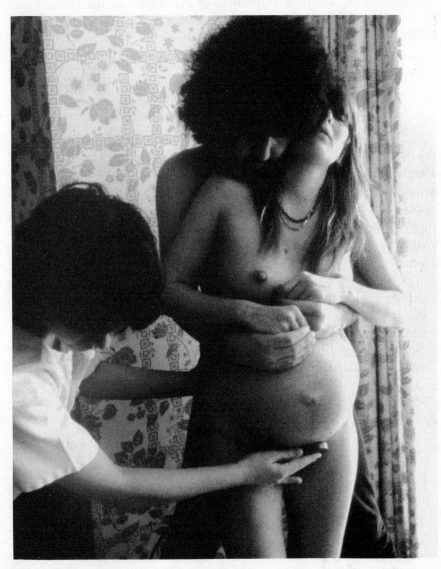

The midwife uses a hand-held monitor to listen to the baby's heartbeat.

the contractions; they feel a need for the close bodily contact of another person, often another woman. If you prefer to be alone during labor, with partner and midwife nearby in another room, you may like to stand and lean forward against the wall during contractions, doing a seated squat on a low stool in between them.

> *"Later in the afternoon Kurt and I went walking alone. I just wanted to hold him during the contractions. I felt such strength from him. When I came into the house the contractions were very strong, and I held Kurt around the neck and hung down. Until the final stage of my labor I had not related much to Kurt, finding I needed the soft quality of a woman, but at the end it was wonderful to have his support, both mental and physical."*

Squatting

This is the physiologically most efficient position for labor and birth. It can be very useful at any stage of labor, particularly if you wish to speed things up. Your pelvis is at its most open, gravity is helping, and contractions are intensified due to increased pressure from the baby's head on the cervix. Some women find this the most comfortable posture.

You may squat during contractions or in between them. Squatting during contractions will probably make them feel much stronger. In between, it will help to widen your pelvis and encourage the baby's descent.

Squatting can tire you out, if you're not careful. It is important to rest completely in between contractions. Use the support of another person or a stool, a pile of big, heavy books, or a firm cushion to make yourself as comfortable as possible.

> *"I continued to squat through contractions. This position seemed most natural and comfortable to me, especially when I spread my knees as wide apart as I could and squirmed from side to side, all the while trying to keep my breathing slow and deep, concentrating on breathing out."*

Some women find the intensity of the contractions while squatting overwhelming. They prefer to use other supported upright positions that are less tiring, such as kneeling forward over a beanbag chair, and to reserve squatting until the very end.

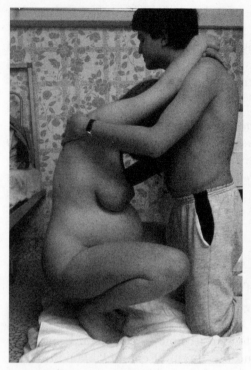

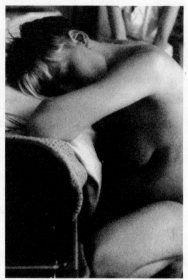

Squatting while leaning forward onto a bed

Supported squatting in labor

Sitting

Sitting upright in labor—on a chair, on a bed, or on the floor—is very comfortable for most women. The contractions are not as intense as with squatting, but they are usually more manageable and are still gravity-effective. It is easy to rest between contractions by leaning forward onto a soft beanbag chair, a cushion, or a bed.

> *"I found that the toilet seat was a very comfortable place because it supported me while leaving my pelvic floor free."*

Kneeling

Most women find that, as labor intensifies and advances to the last part of the first stage (6 to 10 centimeters dilation), kneeling, upright or on all fours, is the most comfortable position. Indeed, many women kneel

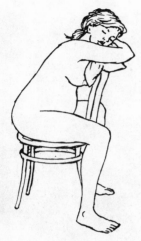

Sitting astride a chair, facing
backwards

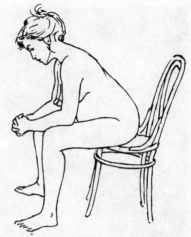

Sitting on a chair leaning forward.
This can also be done on the toilet.

throughout labor. Some find it helpful to move the pelvis rhythmically during contractions, either rotating or rocking, as they kneel. Between contractions, one can relax totally in the kneeling position with the body supported by cushions or a beanbag chair.

"I went on all fours, where I found that a gentle rocking motion eased the pain. My partner rubbed the lower part of my back almost continuously."

The kneeling positions are especially helpful if you have "back labor" or if the baby is lying in a posterior position (see chapter 7). Rhythmic rotation or spontaneous movement of the pelvis can help the baby to turn to the more usual anterior position.

You may kneel with your trunk upright, or you may prefer to lean forward onto a firm pile of cushions or piece of furniture. Make sure that the angle of your trunk is nearly vertical to allow gravity to assist you. Place something soft under your knees, as they can get quite sore if you kneel for a long time on a hard surface. A cushion or a foam-rubber mat (about 2 inches thick) is most helpful.

"When the contractions became much stronger I knelt against the beanbag and rotated my hips. It really did help, in fact, it seemed the most natural thing to do!"

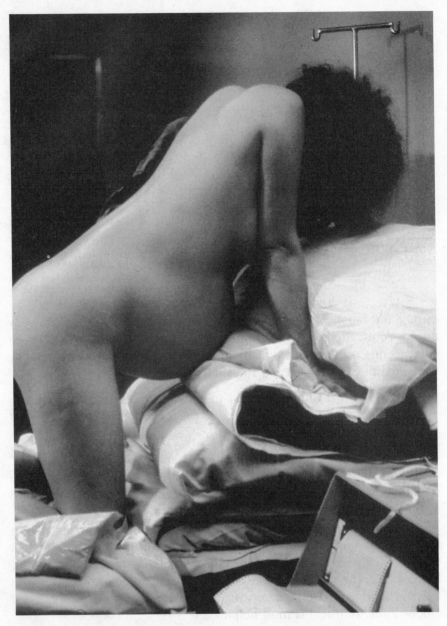

When you kneel upright, gravity helps the baby descend.

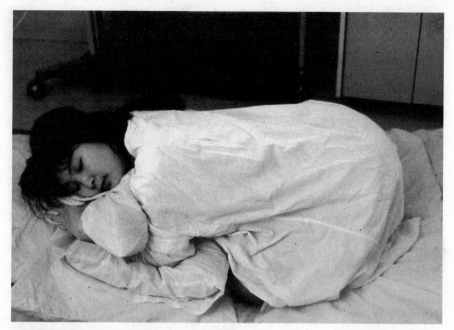

Resting between contractions

If labor is progressing rapidly, you could use a more horizontal kneeling position if you wish to slow things down a little. The less vertical and more horizontal your upper body, the slower the contractions, as the downward force of gravity on the cervix lessens. In the case of a very fast labor, the knee-chest position (see page 131) will help to slow down the contractions and make them less overwhelming.

> *"I knew my baby was coming really fast, and I wanted to slow it down. I was kneeling on the floor, so I put my head down onto the floor and my bottom up in the air."*

Used in many religions as a position for prayer, kneeling can help you turn your awareness inwards. This way you can focus your attention on the contractions rather than on what is going on around you.

Half-kneeling and half-squatting is a good position to use combined with kneeling. It is easier than squatting. Change legs for each contraction, and rock forwards and backwards during contractions. This posture assists the dilation and may ease backache.

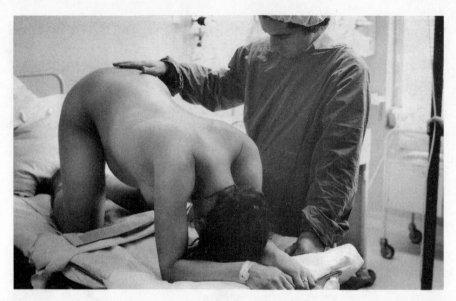

*Kneeling head down is helpful
during intense contractions.*

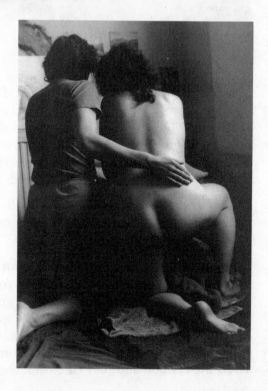

*Half-kneeling, half-squatting
during labor*

"I found the half-kneeling position comfortable; in fact, it was during a strong contraction in this position that the waters broke, and I found that a great relief."

Side-lying

If you wish to lie down during the first stage, it is preferable to do so on your side, with your trunk well propped up by cushions and perhaps a pillow under one knee. You can come up onto all fours if the contractions feel too uncomfortable, then lie down again to rest in between.

TRANSITION

I once heard a midwife explain to a woman in labor that the first stage was rather like climbing a high mountain; at the end of the steep incline one reaches a very difficult craggy bit. Although the top and the view down the other side are close at hand, one can lose sight of the end and fall into despair, struggling with these last difficult contractions.

This is an apt description of transition. It is like a bridge between the last dilating contractions and the beginning of the bearing down in the second stage. Transition can last for as little as a few seconds or as long as two or three hours or more. It is more common to have a long transition with a first than with a later birth.

Transition is a very sensitive time. While the final opening is taking

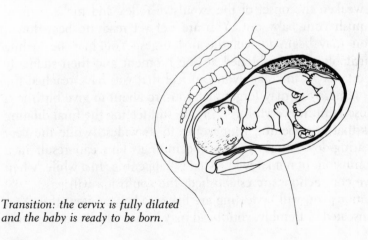

Transition: the cervix is fully dilated and the baby is ready to be born.

place, you are on the threshold of giving birth. As in the moment before orgasm, you will need to be without disturbance or distraction to let go to the involuntary impulses that will bring your baby to birth.

What Happens to Your Baby

Your baby descends a little further into the pelvic canal during transition. The uterus has been drawn up around the baby's head, so that he or she begins to move out of the uterus. Your baby is ready to be born.

What Happens to You

Your contractions are coming fast and furious with very short intervals between them. Your cervix is probably 8 to 9 centimeters dilated, but that last centimeter or two may be very slow to open. A common occurrence at this stage is what is known as an anterior lip—the front rim, or lip, of the cervix still needs to be taken up before the way is clear to bear down and push your baby out.

How You Feel

This is not easy to describe! Most women find transition the most trying part of labor. There you are, wide open and completely vulnerable. It is too late to take any drugs—and very unwise to do so, because at this stage they could weaken the onset of the expulsive reflex and make it more difficult to push your baby out. You are not yet ready to bear down, although you may begin to feel the first urges. You may be feeling desperate, irritable, and frightened at one moment and then suddenly blissful or ecstatic. At this stage you can feel that you have reached the end of your tether; you may forget that you are about to give birth to a baby, and lose faith in everything. You are still feeling the final dilating contractions that are opening your womb to its widest, while the very different bearing-down urges may be beginning. This can result in a feeling of confusion, of not knowing what is happening. In a while, when the expulsive contractions are established, the confusion will pass.

The sensations you will be feeling are likely to be very powerful. You may feel nauseated or trembly; your head may be hot while your feet may be cold. The important thing to remember is that it will all pass, and that the long haul of the first stage is almost over. Most women appear to be in a kind of trance at this stage of labor.

"I squatted or knelt on the mattress supported on both sides by my friend and my husband, and I had a rather short and extremely relaxed transition period. I believe I even slept for a spell."

"This was the most difficult part as I didn't realize I was in transition and felt I wanted to push. I was worried, as this seemed far too early to want to push. I knelt forward on the cushions. I found that eye contact with my husband was important at this stage. When I felt panic during transition my husband breathed with me to slow my breathing down. This immediately brought me back in control."

It is common to feel frightened during transition—after all, you are about to give birth, and to see your baby for the first time! Many women feel that they cannot do it, or even that they may split apart or die. This irrational fear is sometimes not even conscious. Michel Odent calls it "physiological fear"; he believes that this fear just before giving birth has a useful function in raising the level of adrenaline. Whereas earlier in labor adrenaline could inhibit the work of the endorphins, now it has a useful function in helping to trigger the involuntary expulsive reflex of the second stage, which Odent calls "the fetus ejection reflex." He believes the attendants should not overly reassure or disturb the mother at this stage. In his observations, if she is left more or less alone to experience this fear, a quick and efficient expulsive reflex usually follows.[2,3]

During transition you may feel very thirsty. This unusual thirst, together with the dilation of the pupils that is common in transition, is a sign of an increase in adrenaline. It is helpful to take sips of water, or to suck on a natural sponge—women often experience a primitive sucking reflex during labor.

Bathe your face with a face cloth rinsed out in cold water to refresh yourself between contractions.

For some women, being completely alone in a darkened room can help to get through this stage. Others need sensitive, nonintrusive support.

"My mother-in-law gave me sips of warm water with a little honey added and washed my hands and face. Another thing that I found very comforting and refreshing during the whole labor was to suck upon a wet sponge."

Breathing for Transition

Keep up your deep breathing, concentrating on the exhalations to help you relax. If your breathing naturally becomes shallower, then follow your own instincts. Some women need to shout out, moan, curse, or make a lot of noise at this stage of the labor to help relieve pain, whereas others need to be very quiet. It is most important that you should not be disturbed or distracted unnecessarily. Peace and quiet will help you to sink deeply inwards at this stage.

"The thing I found a tremendous help and relief was making a furious grunting, squealing noise at the height of each pain. It was a way of controlling myself, both physically and mentally."

"The contractions were very powerful, and I began to feel extremely tired between them. I flopped forward onto two big cushions and felt as though I could sleep even for a few moments between contractions. The conservation of energy was simply wonderful. I didn't even speak when spoken to."

Positions for Transition

Once again, follow your own instincts and use any position you have found helpful so far.

The kneeling position is the one most women prefer during transition. Use a good firm pile of cushions, or else lean forward onto another person, so that you can rest completely supported in the short breaks between contractions. Allow yourself to sink into a state of deep relaxation. You may like to sit back on your heels sometimes and stretch your arms up between contractions.

If you have a very long transition, try changing positions from time to time—sit upright on the edge of the bed or on a chair, stand up, walk slowly, or lie on your side well propped up by cushions. Many women find it helpful to sit on the toilet in transition.

Knee-Chest Position for an Anterior Lip

Although it is not usually necessary, your nurse or midwife may want to examine you internally at this stage to see if you are fully dilated. If she cannot feel the cervix at all, you are ready to bear down and give birth to your baby. If, however, she can still feel a little rim of cervix in front of the baby's head—an anterior lip—she may advise you to wait until the lip has gone, especially if it is starting to swell.

Resisting the urge to bear down can be very difficult. It will help you to go into the knee-chest position, with your head lower than your bottom. This position brings the baby forward and reduces pressure on the cervix. Move your hips a little during contractions to assist the dilation. The lip will probably have gone after a few contractions. If the urge to bear down is very strong, then try blowing in short bursts (rather than one long sustained breath) when you have the urge, as if you are blowing out a candle three feet away. Don't try this for more than 15 minutes, however, as resisting the pushing urge for too long may weaken the contractions. If the urge to bear down is irresistible, the lip will probably move out of the way with your expulsive efforts.

> *"Billie felt an anterior lip, and I went into knee-chest position to counteract the strong pushing urge. Fortunately, after only a few contractions and blowing it went, and I got up."*

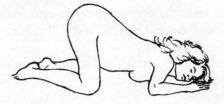

The knee-chest position is useful for slowing down strong contractions.

THE SECOND STAGE OF LABOR

The second stage begins when your baby's head makes contact with the pelvic floor. This stimulates the onset of the expulsive reflex, which brings your baby through the curved birth canal. The head "crowns" when it reaches the perineum, and then your baby is born.

What Happens to Your Baby

After full dilation of the cervix, your baby's head is free of the uterus, and the contractions bring your child's head to the middle of the pelvic canal. At this point the head meets the pelvic floor. Descent continues, and there is further rotation as the head comes down under the pubic bone in front. This may take time. The rotation is usually complete before the back of the head reaches your vulva, although it may still be turning as it is born. Then the crown of your child's head appears, stretching your vaginal opening. With further contractions the face sweeps under your perineum. The body rotates; first one shoulder and then the other emerges. Then the child's body quickly slips out.

In passing through the pelvis, your child's head has been subjected to considerable pressure. That the descent occurs without damage to the head is possible because the bones are soft and because the edges of the skull bones are not yet fused, so they can overlap slightly. Your baby's head may seem slightly pointed in shape after birth due to this "molding," but it will soon round out.

During the delivery, and for some minutes after, your child still receives oxygen from the placenta, through the umbilical cord. After the birth of the head the baby may take a first breath of air, but a short time will pass before full breathing is established. The cord should not be cut until it stops pulsating.

Using upright positions for the second stage will help to ensure that your baby is getting as much oxygen as he or she needs and will minimize the pressure on the baby's head.

What Happens to You

You begin the second stage fully dilated and ready to give birth to your baby. Your uterus begins to contract powerfully from above to push the baby down through the curved birth canal, under the pubic arch, and onto the pelvic floor. The expulsive contractions may start before you are fully dilated, or they may begin 5 to 10 minutes or longer after dilation is complete. After a long transition, your uterus may need to rest. If you have a gap when nothing happens, make the most of it by resting in readiness for the birth. Occasionally this gap can last quite a long time,

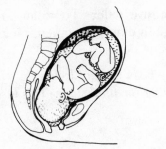

Early second stage

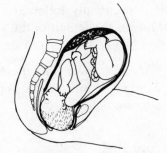

Crowning

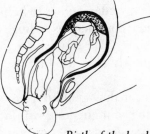

Birth of the head

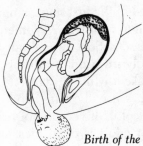

Birth of the shoulders

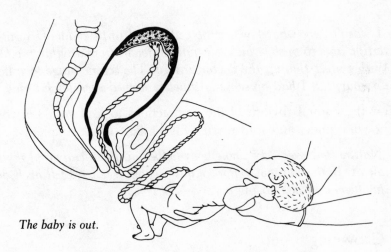

The baby is out.

but it is eventually followed by the expulsive reflex. There are great variations in the length of the second stage in different women, ranging between two and three minutes and as many hours.

"My cervix was fully dilated, but my body did not feel quite ready to push. It was resting, getting ready for the final stage. This lasted over an hour."

How You Feel

These contractions feel quite different from those of the first stage. The intervals between them are generally longer. Even if you feel very tired at the end of the first stage, a new rush of energy often comes to help you give birth to your baby. Women describe these contractions as huge tidal waves of sensation throughout the whole body. The expulsive reflex is completely involuntary. It may come on quickly after the first stage, or it may take a while to start.

There is usually a tremendous urge to bear down, although not all women feel it. If you do not resist this feeling, but go along with it, the muscular effort is often pleasurable. Pressure builds up enormously at this stage, and any resistance to the expulsive effort causes discomfort and pain.

"I wasn't sure what I was supposed to feel until suddenly I got a terrific urge to push, which felt quite different from anything so far. With perfect timing, the doctor arrived. The second stage took half an hour, but I had no sense of time. It seemed very quick to me."

Allow the natural rhythm of the contractions to lead you. Let your body be your guide, and your uterus will do its job.

"Nature took over. My whole body helped automatically and rhythmically in the enormous effort of pushing out a baby. I felt his head, shoulders and body being born."

The Crowning

Your baby's head and neck will extend backwards as they pass under the pubic bone and through the curve of the birth canal. When the crown of the baby's head begins to show through your vagina it is time to get into a suitable position for the birth of the baby (see page 139). You might try feeling the head with your hand as it descends. This first contact with your baby is memorable, and helps you to feel exactly what is happening.

To be born, your child will have to pass through your pelvic floor. In view of its action in childbirth, the pelvic floor can be regarded as consisting of two parts—the front, pubic part and the back, sacral part. The sacral part, attached to your ischial tuberosities (sitting bones), coccyx, and sacrum, is known as the perineum.

To be free to move backwards when the baby is born, the sacral area of the pelvic floor, or perineum, must be relaxed. The position of your body at this stage is all-important. If you are lying on your back, your sacrum is not free to move backwards, and the back, sacral part of your pelvic floor is not in a relaxed state. This forces your child's head to press forward towards the bony sub-pubic arch, instead of backwards towards your sacrum and coccyx, which are mobile and extendable. But if you are squatting, kneeling, or standing, the position of your pelvis is altered, so your sacrum and coccyx extend backwards. When your child's head presses against your perineum, it will be relaxed and able to give as much as possible.

The crowning ends with the birth of the baby. You may have one contraction when your baby's head is born, and then a pause before the next contraction, when the rest of the body emerges. Alternatively, the baby may be born in one contraction. Once the head is born, your baby will turn, so that the shoulders line up with the widest diameter of the pelvic outlet. Then one shoulder will be born, and the baby will continue turning as the other shoulder emerges. Finally the whole body will slip out.

How You Feel

At this stage, the sensations you feel are very intense—a unique mixture of pain and ecstasy. At the end of the crowning, when the head is about to be born and the perineal tissues stretch to their maximum, you may have a feeling of acute stretching and burning—similar to how it feels when you pull at the corners of your mouth with your fingers—mingled with the total body sensation of the contractions. However, as soon as you give birth to the head, which is the widest part of the baby's body, you feel tremendously relieved. If the baby is broad-shouldered, you will feel further stretching as first one shoulder and then the other is born, but as your baby's body slithers out into the world the sensations are usually very pleasurable and often described as totally orgasmic.

"The baby came out gradually and easily without any pushing from me. I felt a burning sensation in my perineum as he was being born and, on checking, I didn't even have a tear."

"I felt an incredible presence in the room, and feelings were high. The pain was almost unbearable, yet now the overpowering urge to bear down was there. It was one of the most powerful bodily sensations I think I have ever had, and soon I saw her head in the mirror, a patch of thick black hair. With an extraordinary release of energy her head came out, but the energy to push was so strong that immediately after her whole body shot out. I felt the utmost release and joy and wonder and thankfulness. Words cannot adequately express that feeling at the moment of birth. I wanted to cry and shout for joy."

Breathing for the Second Stage

When you are in an upright squatting or kneeling position, your breathing can be spontaneous. You may find it helpful, however, to start off each contraction by focusing on your exhalation, as you give in to the powerful urges coming from inside your body.

Breathe deeply, concentrating on the out-breath, as you feel the contraction coming on. You will probably feel an uncontrollable desire to push downwards at the peak of the contraction, as your uterus presses down to expel your baby. The urge to bear down is similar to the way you feel when you defecate. It is best not to tense up against the contractions, as this could be very painful. Just push when you feel like it, following the urge, and holding your breath for short intervals, if you like. You need not try to practice this ahead of time; your body will know what to do when the time comes.

Some nurses and doctors still give a mother orders to hold her breath and push—orders that may not coincide with her own urges. This practice became common when mothers lay on their backs and pushed strenuously so the baby could negotiate the pelvic canal "uphill," in defiance of gravity. However, there is no advantage to pushing strenuously and holding your breath for long periods, especially when you are upright. In fact, this could reduce the supply of oxygen to your baby. Instead, allow your natural urges to lead you.

If the second stage is difficult, choose the most gravity-effective position—the standing squat—and continue breathing spontaneously, pushing only when you feel the urge. If you don't get anywhere like this, however, you should ask your nurse or midwife to guide you in pushing more actively.

Feel free to let out sound as you give birth to your baby. A distinctive "birth cry" is natural and instinctive during the second stage, particularly as the baby is actually coming out. It is best not to resist the urge to cry out, as it is nature's way of assisting you to give birth. The release of tension in your vocal cords stimulates a similar release in your pelvic floor muscles. Women often say that when they screamed during the second stage they felt no pain at all.

At the crowning of your baby's head, your attendant may advise you not to push too hard, or to pant, since holding back at this time will lessen the chances of a perineal tear. Some women find this guidance helpful, but others prefer to totally let go—pushing and resting when they want, and making as much sound as they want. You can give birth as loudly and powerfully, or as softly and gently, as you like. You'll discover your preference only when the time comes.

> *"I squatted on the bed supported by the midwife and my husband and felt my baby emerging. I put my arms under me, and, feeling the head, I let out an unearthly moan, letting the baby slide into my hand. She was warm, creamy, smoother and softer than anything I had ever touched."*

Whichever your approach to giving birth, keep in harmony with the rhythmic sensations you are feeling. Surrender to what your body is telling you.

> *"During the one and a half hours of second stage, I was squatting on the floor almost the whole time, occasionally standing. I felt as comfortable as I could imagine being in labor, and the position, being well supported, enabled me to control my breathing and work with the expulsive contractions as much as possible. I also had a really good view of the emerging head in a mirror propped up in front of me. I gave birth to the baby in the same squatting position."*

Positions for the Second Stage

Your posture makes all the difference to the length and efficiency of the second stage. You will make your child's descent easier if you use upright positions, which allow gravity to help in the safe delivery of your child. Any standing, sitting, kneeling, or squatting position is fine until the baby's head crowns. Then you need to get into a suitable position for the birth.

To understand the advantage of being upright, try this:

1. Squat down on your toes. Breathe in, and tighten your pelvic floor. Hold for a second, and then relax your pelvic floor slowly as you breathe out. Repeat several times.

2. Now try the same thing lying on your back with a pillow under your head. You will probably find that in this position the movement of your perineum is much weaker, and it is more difficult to relax the pelvic floor muscles.

3. Try it again squatting and compare the difference when gravity helps the pelvic floor to relax.

The fit between your child's head and your pelvis is so close that the smallest increase in the size of your pelvis is significant. To understand this:

1. Squat down on your toes and spread your knees apart. Close your eyes, and concentrate on the opening of your pelvis. It is open at its widest in this position, and your sacrum and coccyx are free to move if your child is passing through your pelvic outlet.

2. Now try the semireclining position. Place a few pillows on the floor or against a wall, and lie on your back so your trunk is at an angle of about 15° to the floor. Place your hand under your back, and feel how the whole weight of your body, your uterus, and your baby is lying on your sacrum, which is closed to its maximum. Research suggests that you are losing a significant percentage—up to one-third—of the possible opening (see chapter 1).

When you recline, the weight of your uterus also presses down on the large internal blood vessels in your abdomen, which reduces the supply of oxygen to your baby and is likely to induce fetal distress. Your uterus tilts forward when it contracts. When you are in the semireclining position, it must work against the force of gravity. This makes contractions more painful and less effective.

"On one occasion I was lying on my back to enable Jane to examine me. Unfortunately, I had a contraction while in this position. It was extremely painful, and I would not like to repeat the experience."

Your coccyx is designed to move out of the way as your baby's head descends. Sitting on your coccyx during birth restricts the pelvic outlet and can also lead to dislocation of the coccyx, which can be extremely painful for months after the birth.

These are some of the reasons that women who have the freedom to choose their own positions for delivery rarely choose to semirecline, much less to lie flat on their backs. (In one year at Pithiviers, for instance, only two out of 898 women chose to lie down.)

Each upright position has certain advantages. You will discover which position works best for you at the time. Try them out with your partner in the weeks before the birth so your body will know all the possibilities. Of course, the room and circumstances in which you give birth may limit the positions you can choose. The room should ideally contain little furniture so that you can freely discover the right posture. However, it is possible to use upright birth positions on a bed as well as on the floor (see chapter 7).

Unless the second stage is very short, it is likely that you will change positions—standing and squatting, or squatting and kneeling, or kneeling and sitting up—as your baby descends. It is helpful to have two people nearby to help support you.

Sitting on the toilet may be helpful as the baby descends. Once the head crowns and you feel the baby is coming, of course, it is time to get into a suitable position for the birth.

Many women make the mistake of starting to squat too early. Unless you are very used to squatting and find it restful, you may become tired if you squat too soon in the second stage. Any upright position will do until the head of the baby crowns, and then it is time to use the birth position. If the second stage is very rapid, you will probably feel like being on all fours, where you can remain for the birth. If the second stage is slow, using the hanging squat (see page 140) for a few contractions may help to bring the baby's head down faster.

Supported Squatting

Because it makes optimum use of gravity, the supported standing squat is the most efficient position for the rapid descent of the baby. You stand or walk in between contractions, but as a contraction comes on, your knees bend and you may feel the need to hold on to something. You can hold your partner around the shoulders (in the "hanging squat"), or your partner can support you from behind, while you let go of your weight and surrender to the force of the contraction. After the contraction passes you move freely until the next one, when you are supported again.

Once you have the position right, relax completely against your partner's body. Allow your weight to drop as you go down into a squat, but keep your feet flat, if possible, so that they carry some of your weight. Relax your neck, and rest your head back against your partner's body.

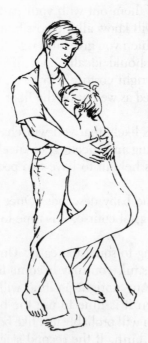

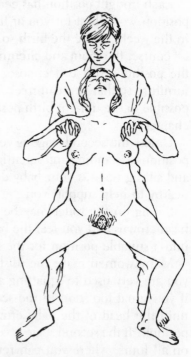

The hanging squat: facing her partner, the mother places her arms around his neck, allowing herself to hang. This position helps the baby to descend.

The supported standing squat: the partner stands behind the mother, holding her under her arms.

Then, with your legs apart and your pelvis heavy, let go to the powerful contractions that bring the baby to birth.

The standing squat has several advantages.

In this position your pelvis is wide open, and you have maximum help from gravity. The upward force of the supporter's body acts as a counterbalance to the downward force of the contractions. The second stage tends to be quickest in this posture; the baby usually comes out in one contraction after the crowning. This is a great advantage if the second stage has been long or difficult; or if there is a difficult presentation (posterior or breech), a big baby, or any suspicion of distress (which is less likely if the labor has been active). This position allows you great freedom to act instinctively—to surrender to your natural urges.

Once the baby is born, the midwife can place him or her safely down in front of you, on an absorbent towel. Then sit down to welcome your baby!

> *"With the first urges to bear down I searched for a posture to help me do so. The best one was with my husband holding me up from behind with his arms passing under mine while I just let myself hang loose. It was not only comfortable for me, but feeling his physical strength revived my now tired body, and it also gave us both a sense of bonding. The bearing down happened on its own, and in just four pushes our baby was out: a beautiful, slippery, gurgly little girl."*

Sitting upright after the birth allows you to hold the baby at just the right angle to breastfeed easily. (When you lie back, your breast tends to slip down sideways, and it's more difficult for the baby to latch on.) This first loving contact—skin to skin and eye to eye—between you and your baby stimulates the production of hormones that cause contraction of the uterus and the separation of the placenta in the third stage.

A bowl of warm water can be placed between your legs so that you can bathe your baby, if you like, before the placenta is delivered or the umbilical cord is cut. Alternatively, you and the baby can bathe together in the bathtub a little later, after the placenta is delivered.

> *"He stared intently at me and then started to suck at my breast. The cord was left attaching us until it stopped pulsing and was white. There was no feeling of separation, only continuation and deep joy and contentment. Everything felt right, and I felt wonderful, not at all tired."*

TIPS FOR THE PARTNER

The supporting position becomes easy if you practice it a little on your own. Even if you are small, once you have the dynamics right you'll be able to support a large and heavy woman with little strain or effort. If you have a weak back or any spinal problems, you should use a chair (see page 149).

It is best to be without socks and shoes. Place your feet two to three feet apart. Bend your knees, and tighten the muscles of your thighs and buttocks, leaning back just a little so that her weight is carried against your pelvis. Keep your back straight; resist the temptation to bend forward, as this would strain your lower back. Keep your arms and shoulders relaxed so that your thighs provide the supporting strength while your upper body remains more or less free from tension.

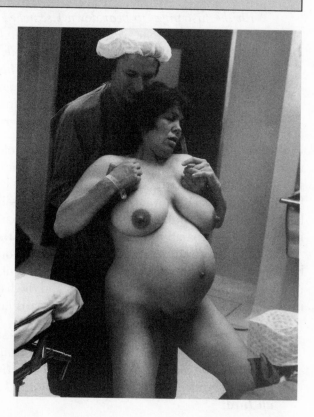

The baby's head crowns, and the mother settles into the supported standing squat, ready for the birth.

Keeping your knees bent, ground yourself by breathing deeply. Try exhaling "through the soles of your feet."

Once your feet and lower body are in position, you are ready to take your partner's weight. Sometimes when the mother stays in the kneeling position to bear down, the baby's head can take a long time to descend. It may appear on the perineum, then disappear back inside between contractions. In such a case it may be practical for the mother to use a more upright position, so that gravity can help the baby's head to crown and to be born. You can suggest this to the mother tactfully between contractions, pointing out that she may make the baby's passage easier by getting into a more upright position. Then very slowly help her up from behind, as illustrated, giving her time to come gradually to a kneeling position, then, one leg at a time, to standing, and then to lower herself into a standing squat. Keeping your shoulders

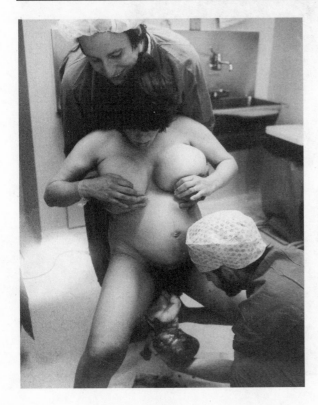

The baby is born in one contraction.

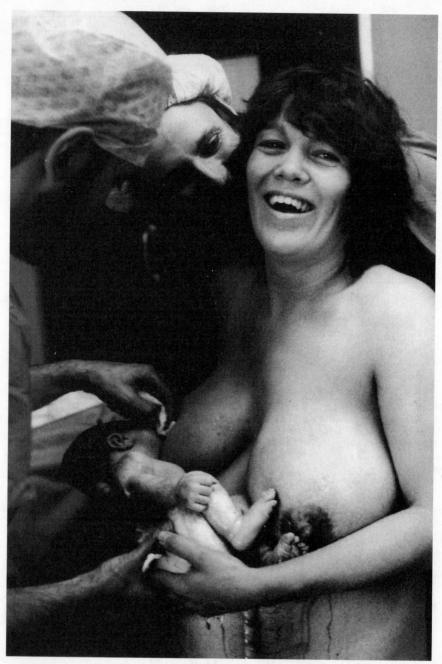

Moments after the birth

TIPS FOR THE PARTNER (cont.)

and upper arms relaxed, pass your hands under her arms with your palms uppermost. She can put her hands on top of yours, palms together, linking her fingers with yours or not, as she prefers. Alternatively, she can make fists with her thumbs up, and you can grasp her thumbs.

Keep your arms and hands as relaxed as possible; let her hold on to you, rather than vice versa. It is a good idea to have a beanbag chair or bed behind your legs, as your partner might drop down very low as the baby is being born. You could then squat on the beanbag chair, and she could squat between your legs.

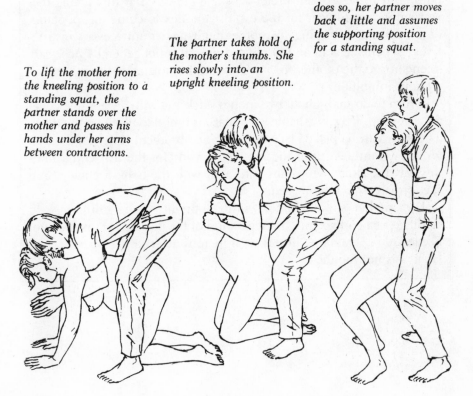

Taking her time, the mother stands up. As she does so, her partner moves back a little and assumes the supporting position for a standing squat.

The partner takes hold of the mother's thumbs. She rises slowly into an upright kneeling position.

To lift the mother from the kneeling position to a standing squat, the partner stands over the mother and passes his hands under her arms between contractions.

TIPS FOR THE ATTENDANT

Supporting the mother in a standing squat is hard work, so it is sensible to use this position only once the head begins to crown, when you can expect the baby to be born in the next few contractions. If descent of the head is slow, however, the hanging squat may be used before crowning to help the head to come down.

A clean sheet covered with an absorbent towel or disposable pad can be placed between the mother's legs to receive the baby. There is usually no need to guard the perineum, as the baby is usually born quite quickly from this position. If the final stage is slow, however, a warm compress held against the perineum will help to prevent tearing and will be soothing for the mother.

Usually the mother does best without any instructions at all; she simply surrenders to her body's urges and cries out as the baby is being born. But some women prefer sensitive guidance at this point. It is very important to wait for the expulsive reflex to come on spontaneously, without disturbing the mother or giving her unnecessary instructions. When she is in an upright position, it is not generally necessary to encourage the mother to "push" but rather to enable her to "let go" without inhibition.

A firm foam mat, about two inches thick and with a washable cover (or a nonslip, light, washable yoga mat), is useful to place on the floor. The baby can be placed face down on an absorbent towel on the mat for a few minutes, until the mother is ready for the first contact. In this way the fluids will drain naturally, with the help of gravity, and suction is very rarely needed.

The mother should remain sitting upright in the third stage to facilitate first contact and the separation of the placenta. Pitocin is not needed to facilitate the third stage if there is no excessive bleeding and labor was not induced.

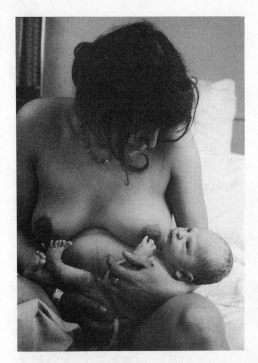

The mother sits upright on a hospital delivery bed moments after squatting on the bed to give birth. In this position she enjoys free contact with her baby. The baby opens his eyes, and first eye contact takes place.

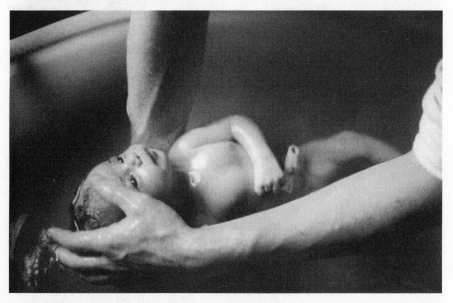

The baby is bathed soon after birth.

Squatting with Two Supporters

Full squatting may be ideal for the woman who can squat easily or has practiced squatting throughout her pregnancy. The pelvis is wide open, and gravity helps the baby to descend. Since the pelvic floor muscles are relaxed, the baby's head can pass through them easily, so tearing is prevented.

During the contraction the mother squats down on the floor. Her two

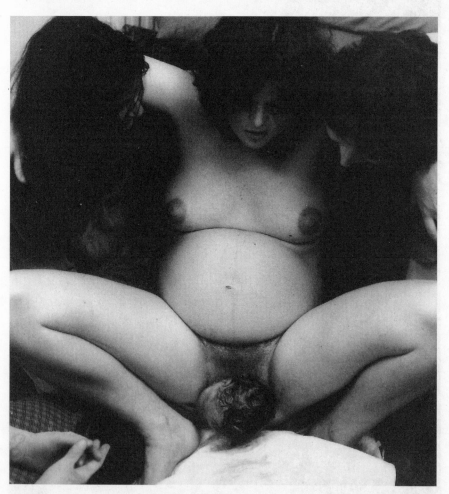

Squatting with two supporters. The midwife waits for the baby to emerge with the next contraction.

supporters kneel on either side of her, each placing one knee just under her buttocks. She can then put one arm around the shoulders of each supporter who, in turn, can put one arm each around her back. Between contractions she can stand up or get onto all fours.

It is important that the supporters are comfortable kneeling. It helps to place a cushion between the calves and buttocks or under the knees.

In this position the mother is free to look down and watch her baby being born in a completely relaxed, supported squat. She can also use her own hands to feel the baby's head descending, to help ease the perineal tissues, and to hold the baby as he or she is born. Some women have a strong instinct to do this themselves.

From this position, it is easy to stand up or move to the all-fours positions.

When the mother is in this full squatting position, the baby, unassisted, will slip out between the mother's legs and land safely in front of her, face downwards. She can then lift up the baby herself.

This position also allows the fluids from the uterus to drain, rather than to partially "pool" in the uterus, as they would if the mother were lying down.

After the birth, the mother can sit down on the floor with her trunk upright. It is much easier for the mother to handle the baby, and for the baby to find the breast, if the mother is upright.

> *"For the second stage I squatted, standing up in between contractions to stretch my legs. I felt marvelous—confident, in control—during this stage, which lasted about three-quarters of an hour. The obstetrician, by turning his head for a moment, missed the actual birth. Lara literally sailed out—a totally solo performance—and exercised her vocal cords immediately!"*

Full squatting can also be used to assist delivery of the placenta.

Supported Squatting Using a Chair

A mother can give birth in the full squatting position even with just one supporter. The supporter can sit on a chair or on the edge of a bed, while the mother squats with her body cradled between the supporter's legs, using his or her thighs for support. Many women find this enjoyable and comforting, as well as comfortable. It is best for the supporter to use a firm chair and to sit well forward on it so that the mother can rest against his or her body. This position is ideal if the supporting partner has a weak back.

> "I squatted between Ron's knees as he sat on a chair, and I supported myself on his thighs with my elbows, resting my back in his lap. We looked in the mirror to see our baby's head emerging, then, before the midwife could put her gloves on, all of him was born, and he was placed in my arms to suckle."

The mother might instead like to face the supporting partner as he or she sits on a chair or stool. They hold each other by the wrists with elbows straight as the mother squats, keeping her heels on the floor. This posture is very easy for both mothers and supporters, and it is especially effective in relaxing the perineum.

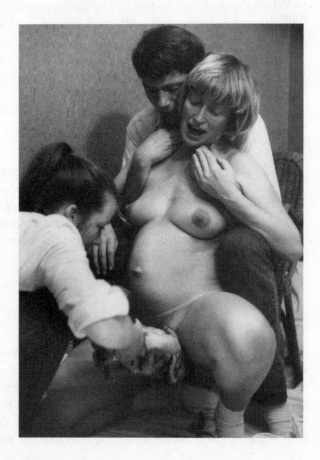

Supported squatting with the partner sitting on a chair. The mother cries out freely as the baby is born.

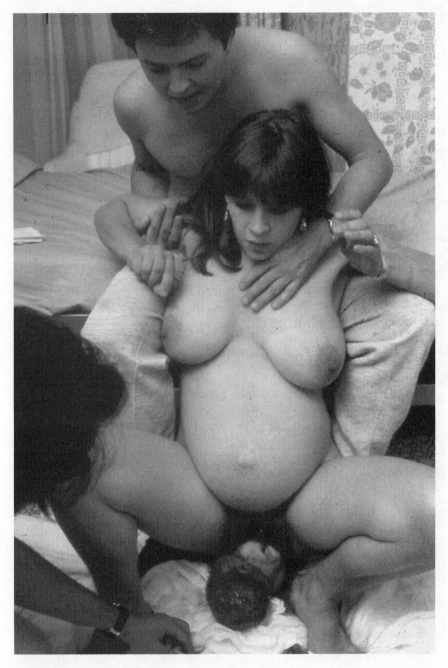

The father sits on the edge of the bed and supports the mother as the baby is born.

Kneeling or All-Fours Position

Here you simply kneel, legs apart, and rest on your hands or against a pile of cushions.

This position, which seems to come very naturally, is often used by women in traditional societies. It is an ideal position if the labor and second stage have been very fast, as it gives you more control and slows the baby's descent a little. If the baby is in a posterior presentation, getting on all fours can relieve pressure on the back and allow you to move your hips gently to help the baby rotate as it descends. Mothers say that this is a very easy way to give birth. In between contractions, you can kneel upright and stretch your arms if you want to.

Once the baby is born and is caught by the doctor or midwife, she can pass the baby through your legs and place it face down in front of you. You can then rest back on your heels or sit down, upright, to see and lift up your baby.

Some mothers instinctively turn over to sit up after delivery in a kneeling position. In this case the doctor or midwife can pass you the baby under one knee as you turn. Often mothers deliver in a half kneeling,

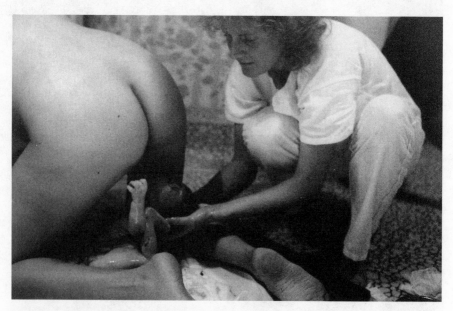

Birth in the all-fours position. The midwife is dressed comfortably so that she too can be active!

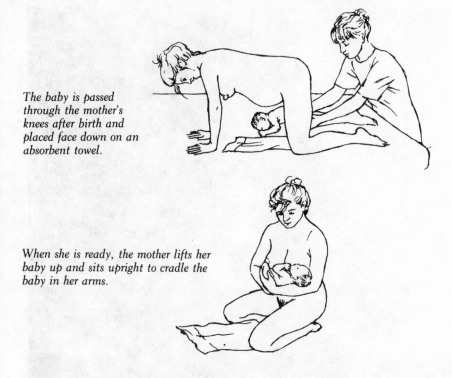

The baby is passed through the mother's knees after birth and placed face down on an absorbent towel.

When she is ready, the mother lifts her baby up and sits upright to cradle the baby in her arms.

half squatting position with one knee up. This position can be useful if you wish to catch the baby yourself.

> "When the second stage began I knelt upright and held on to the top of the bed to push. It took no more than half an hour to push the baby out. I gave birth on all fours then. Without having the cord cut, I turned over and was given the baby. Wonderful! Because I was kneeling and very much in control of how fast the baby was being born, I didn't tear and so was able to walk around quite comfortably shortly after delivery."

Sometimes when a mother kneels in the second stage the baby takes a long time to progress from crowning to birth. The head may appear during contractions, then disappear back in again between. When this is the case, it is best to change to a more vertical squatting position so the birth is not prolonged.

In the case of an unexpectedly very fast second stage, use the knee-chest position to slow down and gain control (see page 131).

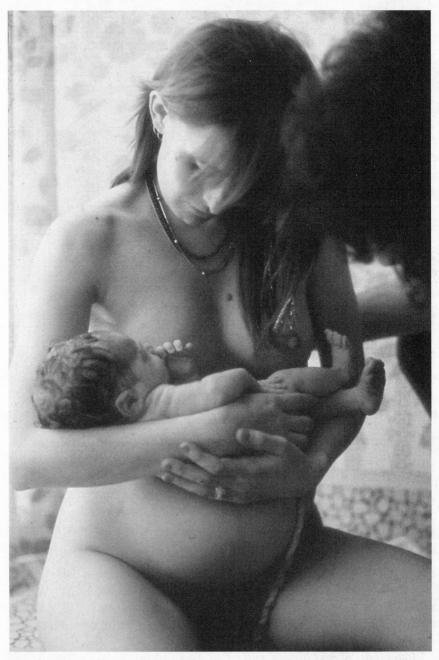

Sitting on her heels after giving birth on all fours, the mother cradles her newborn baby.

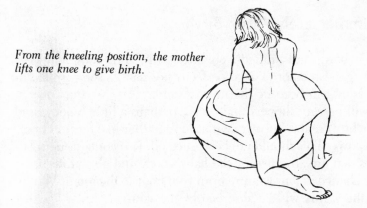

From the kneeling position, the mother lifts one knee to give birth.

Side-Lying

This can sometimes be a useful position for delivery, as it leaves the sacrum free to move. It also offers the same advantages to the attendant—a good view and little bending—as the semireclining position. Since it does not use gravity to full advantage, however, this posture would not be sensible if the second stage is slow. But if the baby is descending without difficulty, you may be comfortable like this:

Lie on your side with your trunk well propped up by pillows, and hook one arm under your knee to support your leg as the baby is born.

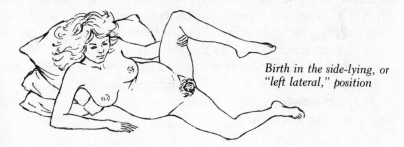

Birth in the side-lying, or "left lateral," position

After the birth, sit upright to hold and put your baby to the breast.

"For me, the right position was simply the one that felt right at the time. This was lying on my left side with my knee drawn to my chest and my hands drawing the opening wider and, at the same time, touching the emerging head. In this way I was able to give a little tactile help in opening my perineum."

The Baby Immediately After Birth

As he or she is born, and immediately after birth, your baby may be a slightly blue or grayish color. This is perfectly normal. As soon as breathing starts the baby will become the normal color.

The baby will be very slippery and moist, perhaps a little bloody, and covered in a white creamy substance that looks rather like cream cheese and is called vernix. This should not be washed off, as it contains nourishing substances that are absorbed by the baby's body and also protects the baby from the change in temperature from your body to the room. Within a few hours, the vernix will be absorbed by the skin.

The baby may be a little wrinkled, too, but after some time its body will become soft and round. Some babies also have fine hairs growing on their ears or other parts of the body at birth; these fall out in the early weeks. The baby's head at first is quite large in proportion to the rest of the body and may be a little pointed, or "molded," from the birth. The genitals are usually a little enlarged as well.

Your baby's eyes will open very soon after the birth—perhaps even before the whole body emerges. The baby will be awake and looking for you! All the baby's senses are acute at this stage. The skin, ears, eyes, and mouth are all receptive to any stimulation. For this first hour or two after birth, the baby will be extremely alert—more so than in the following hours and days—as he or she experiences breathing and sight for the first time. The lungs and digestive system begin to work independently as the baby breathes air and sucks colostrum from your breasts. The baby will need to keep close to you, to the familiar sound of your heartbeat and the warmth of your body, in the early hours, days, and weeks after birth.

If you have twins, you can greet and nurse the firstborn as usual. The first contact between mother and baby will stimulate the contractions that will expel the second twin.

THE THIRD STAGE OF LABOR

After the birth your baby will be in your arms. The rush of emotion will cause your body to secrete hormones that will, after a while, cause your uterus to contract and the placenta to separate from the wall of the uterus. Nature has designed the process to take place quite automatically. As

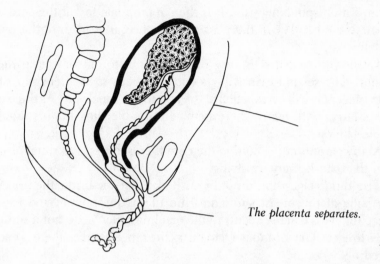

The placenta separates.

your baby comes into contact with your breast or sucks on the nipple, more hormones are secreted, which makes the uterus contract strongly.

Meanwhile, your baby begins to breathe independently through the lungs, and, after 10 to 15 minutes (if not sooner), breathing is fully established and the umbilical cord has stopped pulsating. The placenta and cord continue functioning until breathing is fully established, to guarantee the baby a supply of oxygen and a means of getting rid of carbon dioxide. Particularly in the case of distress or a complication, this supply of oxygen is a natural insurance that the baby will receive sufficient oxygen until he or she is capable of breathing independently.

It is extremely dangerous for a newborn baby to be deprived of oxygen; this can cause brain damage. It is equally dangerous for the baby to have no means of breathing out carbon dioxide. If the baby is still receiving oxygen from the placenta—because the umbilical cord has not been cut prematurely—brain damage is far less likely to occur.

A midwife once told me a story of an unusual situation in a rural area where there was no medical backup and the baby was breathing irregularly for an hour and a half. She left the cord attached, and also gave the baby some oxygen occasionally until the breathing was regular. She observed that the cord continued to function for the entire one and a half hours, and then finally stopped pulsating when the baby no longer needed to breathe through the placenta. The placenta then separated and was delivered, and the baby was in perfect condition.

After the cord has stopped pulsating it becomes completely flaccid and clamps itself spontaneously. It is then appropriate to cut the cord and to separate the baby from the placenta, or one can wait until the placenta is delivered.

Even with twins, it is very important not to cut or clamp the cord earlier. The second twin will probably be born soon after the first, and both placentas will be expelled at the end in the usual way. As the placenta site is larger with twins, there may be more bleeding than is usual with single babies.

Many parents enjoy cutting the cord themselves; it is a ritual of separation that can be very satisfying.

The third stage should not be rushed. After the birth, the suckling of the baby at the breast stimulates the uterus to contract and expel the placenta. This usually occurs in the first hour after birth, but it sometimes takes longer. There is no need to hurry the process unless there is excessive bleeding.

Administering Pitocin to induce contractions of the uterus is rarely necessary if the mother has given birth in an upright position and her baby has not been separated from her. Pitocin may be needed to reduce the risk of postpartum hemorrhage when the mother has been lying down during labor, when she has had an anesthetic or other drug that reduces the ability of the uterus to contract spontaneously, or when she and the baby are separated at birth and the normal hormonal secretion is thus disturbed. When postpartum hemorrhage occurs, Pitocin is very useful in stopping it, but giving birth actively diminishes the chance of such an

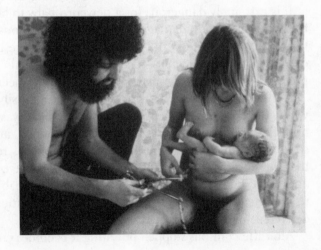

After the placenta has been expelled the umbilical cord is clamped, and then the father cuts it.

occurrence. Pitocin has certain risks that make its use inadvisable when labor and birth have been normal and spontaneous (see page 8), yet it is still given routinely in some hospitals. You may need to talk with your birth attendant in advance about how to avoid it.

When the placenta is separating from the walls of the uterus you will feel the contractions coming on and can then squat to allow the uterus to expel the afterbirth. The placenta is approximately one-sixth the size of the baby and is very soft, so it is much easier to deliver. The sensations women feel as the placenta comes out are very enjoyable—it is like ending on a pleasant and healing note.

"The placenta was born half an hour later. I simply squatted over a dish, and with one gentle push out it came!"

Although it isn't painful, cord traction—pulling on the cord to deliver the placenta—is not usually advisable, as it increases the risk of a fragment of placenta being left behind, which could cause an infection. It also robs you of the pleasure of delivering the placenta spontaneously.

Remember to have a look at the placenta, if you want to. In some societies, extensive rituals surround the disposal of the afterbirth, because it has been part of the baby in the womb and is regarded as having magical properties. Many animals eat the placenta; the hormones it contains help the uterus to contract and return to normal. Now and then, women do the same thing, some cooking it into a stew with wine and mushrooms! Other people take the placenta home in a plastic bag to bury under a favorite tree.

After the birth your doctor or midwife will examine your vagina and perineum to see if you have torn. If you have, or if an episiotomy was done, the doctor will give you a local anesthetic to prevent your feeling any pain, and then stitch up the tear. It is advisable to accept the local anesthesia, even for one stitch, as it poses no danger to the baby, and the stitching can be very painful without it. You can continue to hold your baby while the stitching is being done. It is not necessary to use foot stirrups; in fact, you can probably relax better with your legs apart on the bed, knees bent. Soothing, antiseptic herbal baths will speed the healing of a tear or episiotomy (see page 218).

Your baby will also be examined, and this too can be done while he or she is still in your arms, if you wish. Although labor is over, the third stage is a very important time for you, your partner, and your baby. Your baby is at his or her most alert. You and the baby will be, in a sense, meeting each other for the first time, looking into each other's eyes and sharing your first hours together. After just a few hours your baby will fall asleep; he or she will be sleepy or nursing most of the time in the next week or so.

You need to take your time together, to integrate and share your feelings, and to celebrate the arrival of a new person in your family. This bonding is an essential part of your new relationship. Most of the procedures that need to be done after birth, such as examining the baby in detail, can wait for an hour or so.

Try to spend a few hours together with just your family following the birth. If complications at birth make this impossible, then take the very first opportunity to be alone together in just the same way.

> *"He lay on me for an hour and a half, while my husband and I talked quietly, thoroughly involved in getting to know our new little son. That night we were never separated. The baby calmly looked all around him with a quiet awareness before at last falling asleep. For me those hours will never be forgotten."*

7 | Active Birth at Home or in the Hospital

YOU WILL PROBABLY BE ASKED TO CHOOSE THE PLACE OF birth right at the beginning of your pregnancy, and you may be expected to stay committed to your original choice. But it is not always easy to decide at this time, as you may not know very much about the whole subject, or the options available. Certainly you will not yet know how the pregnancy is to progress, which must influence your final choice. Women, like other mammals, have a powerful "nesting instinct," which usually arises towards the end of the pregnancy. Just as a cat chooses her corner of the house before the kittens are due to arrive, you too may not know where you wish to give birth until closer to the end, though you may have some idea of the kind of setting you would prefer.

When you begin your prenatal care with your doctor, midwife, or clinic, keep open all your options for the birth. In the meantime, explore the possibilities. You may wish to change your doctor for the remainder of your pregnancy, or to choose a hospital that may not be your nearest because you like its approach. It is advisable to pay a visit to any hospital you are considering before committing yourself, to find out about the general approach in the labor ward and whether the staff encourages activity during labor and upright positions for birth. Also find out what happens after the birth, and how long you will be expected to stay before you can go home with your baby. You might prefer to explore the other options available. Remember: You are always entitled to change your mind.

Home or Hospital?

There is no way of removing every risk in childbirth. Although the vast majority of babies are born safely, the final outcome of any birth is always uncertain. Unexpected complications can arise, machines can break down; anyone can make a mistake. There is now plenty of evidence that *in general* it is as safe, if not safer, to have a baby at home as to have it in the hospital, and home usually provides the best conditions for a physiological birth. But different factors, such as your health, your insurance plan, your proximity to a hospital, and whether you have any problems in pregnancy, will help to determine the most appropriate place of birth. The most important thing is to discover all the possibilities, to consider what your priorities are, and then to make a choice that feels right for you. Your instinctive feelings are really important, and they will arise most strongly at the end of your pregnancy. Your choice of birth place may depend upon your choice of birth attendant, or vice versa. Most births in the United States are attended by obstetricians—surgeons who are trained to handle complications, and who are likely to resort to obstetrical interventions. You may instead choose a family practitioner, a physician who provides both obstetrical and newborn care and is trained to view birth as a normal process. Or you may choose one of the growing number of certified nurse-midwives (CNMs). Experts in the normal birth, CNMs may attend deliveries in hospitals, birthing centers, and homes. They sometimes work in group practice with physicians, and they refer women with complications to specialists. Finally, you may prefer a "direct-entry" midwife—a midwife who has entered the profession directly, usually through apprenticeship, rather than going to nursing school first. These midwives specialize in home birth. Their legal status varies from state to state, and your insurance company probably won't pay expenses for a birth attended by a midwife who is unlicensed. But sometimes, for a home birth, there is no alternative. A minority of CNMs and very few physicians attend births at home, because of pressure from hospitals, colleagues, and insurors, and sometimes because of legal restrictions.

If you, like most American women, choose to have your baby in a hospital with an obstetrician, you can still have something like the constant nurturing a midwife provides. You can have an experienced friend or relative, a trained labor support provider, a lay midwife, or a childbirth educator accompany you to the hospital to provide support throughout your labor.

Nowadays many hospitals have special, private birthing rooms that are used for both labor and delivery, and some have alternative birth centers where routines and interventions are greatly reduced. Also available in some areas are freestanding birth centers, which combine the comforts of home with proximity to emergency facilities. See "Resources" for more information on the choices available.

If you have any of the following problems, you may need to have your baby in a hospital.

Preeclampsia

Sometimes called toxemia, this condition can occur when blood pressure rises to dangerous levels. I do not mean the slight rise in blood pressure that is quite common at the end of pregnancy, and that needs careful observation but generally presents no problems. Blood pressure is connected with emotions, and sometimes the excitement of the approaching birth can cause a slight rise. But when the diastolic pressure (the second figure in the reading) rises by 15, you are considered to have hypertension. This can be, though it isn't necessarily, a symptom of preeclampsia. Other symptoms include edema (swelling) and protein in the urine. These can be signs of kidney and liver failure, and may result in premature labor or deprivation of oxygen and nutrients to the baby, and convulsions or coma (eclampsia) in the mother. Fortunately, eclampsia is very rare these days.

Sometimes, with bed rest and good diet, (including plenty of protein), mild preeclampsia will improve. If it doesn't, it may be safest to have the baby in the hospital. With persistent preeclampsia, doctors prefer to induce labor.

If you are confined to bed in pregnancy it will help to get up every few hours to do some relaxing yoga-based exercises for half an hour, and then return to bed.

Breech Presentation

There are more risks involved in this case than in a normal presentation. (See "Unusual Presentations.")

Previous Complications

Not all complications are likely to recur. However, if there were problems with the last birth that could affect this one, you may be better off in the hospital. It is helpful to reflect on what happened last time and discuss the causes with your birth attendant. Sometimes getting a second professional opinion can help you determine whether or not the same problems are likely to recur. For example, if you had a cesarean section for pelvic disproportion, you may need one again (although this is not a certainty). But if the cause of the cesarean was fetal distress, the events are much less likely to be repeated.

Placenta Previa

Sometimes the placenta lies very low in the uterus, close to or covering the cervix. The danger is that the placenta could separate and be born before the baby, which would cause the baby to be cut off from its source of nourishment.

Although women with low-lying placentas usually end up with perfectly normal births, it may be necessary to have help close at hand in case a cesarean is required. (With a full placenta previa, in which the placenta covers the cervix, a cesarean is always necessary.)

Twins

Sometimes twins are born prematurely, so it is important to choose a hospital that has intensive care facilities for newborns. If there are no complications and both babies are a good size at full term, it is certainly possible to have an active birth; the supported standing squat (see page 140) is the best position to use.

As twins tend to be smaller than single babies, birth may in fact be easier. The positions the babies are lying in during labor can affect the outcome. Both babies may be head down; this is the best outlook for twins. However, often the second twin is in a breech position. If this is the case, an active birth is essential, with vigilance on the part of the attendants, to avoid the use of forceps or a cesarean section. Sometimes the second twin lies sideways (transverse) and the doctor can manually turn it head down from the outside before birth.

With an active birth of twins, the first is born using a supported squatting position. If there is time, the mother sits down to welcome the firstborn, whose sucking at the breast stimulates the uterus to contract to expel the second twin.

Since there are two placental sites with twins, bleeding is more than usual, and Pitocin may be needed.

Rh Negative with Antibodies

The rhesus factor is found in the red blood cells. Most people are Rh positive (Rh +); 15 percent are Rh negative (Rh −). If you are Rh − and your mate is Rh +, chances are you are carrying a Rh + baby. If your baby is Rh + and his blood mingles with yours (which sometimes happens during the last three months of pregnancy or at birth), then you will develop antibodies to Rh + blood. You will have blood tests during pregnancy to see if you have any of these antibodies, and at 28 weeks your doctor or midwife will offer you an injection of Rhogam, which can prevent you from developing any. If you forgo the injection and no antibodies develop, there is nothing to be concerned about. Your baby's blood is most likely to mingle with yours at birth (it happens only rarely, anyway), and by the time you may have developed the antibodies the baby will probably be born.

If you do not have a Rhogam injection in pregnancy and a blood sample from the cord shows the baby is Rh +, within 72 hours of the birth you should have a Rhogam injection, which will prevent you from developing antibodies that could affect your next baby. Before this injection was available, Rh − women sometimes had great difficulties, and sometimes their babies needed a complete blood change after birth to clear away the antibodies.

Provided you have no antibodies in your blood, the pregnancy and birth can take place without any cause for concern. If you have antibodies, you will need to deliver in a hospital.

ACTIVE BIRTH AT HOME

"There was a feeling of great calm and peace and relaxation, and we all lay down together in our family bed for the night. It felt so good not to have a separation from either Kurt or David."

There are many advantages to a home birth. In your own home you are the center around which everything else revolves, rather than a patient, dependent on the routines of a large institution. Your attendants come into your home as guests. You can relax in the comfort and security of a familiar atmosphere, with your loved ones around you. The birth is a special event in your family life, a time to celebrate. For the other children in the family, particularly if they are very young, a home birth is of great value, as they can welcome their new brother or sister without having to cope with a separation from you. If all goes well, you may choose to have the children present at the actual birth and, in this way, completely included in the experience.

"As he was born and we were waiting for the cord to stop pulsating, I suddenly became more aware of how wonderful it was, for us all to be together at this time. The girls had witnessed the birth of their brother, a strong bonding experience."

With home birth you have the great advantage of continuity of care, from early pregnancy through labor. There is plenty of time to get to know the midwife or midwives who are going to attend you at the birth, and to discuss your wishes with them in advance. Or you can have the comfort of your own family doctor being present at the birth. Make the most of the many opportunities to discuss what you intend to do with your doctor or midwife. You will approach the birth with more confidence if you feel that you can trust your attendants to support and encourage you to give birth actively. If they are unfamiliar with this book, share it with them as you make plans together.

"The prospect of even a small difficulty ahead suddenly daunted me, and being at home, in loving arms, made it easier for me to protest that I couldn't face it. In the hospital, being geared to fight off interference, I was also fully geared to fight my own weakness, whereas at home it was safe for me to want to give up without risking interventions I would later regret."

At home you can avoid routine hospital practices and the temptation to resort to drugs or other interventions in your weaker moments. You are the only person present in labor, and the birth process can unfold naturally. You can take your time, and you are not subjected to the inconvenience of moving to the hospital, which usually disturbs the rhythm of labor and slows contractions. You can create the ideal environment, use the bathroom whenever you want to, make as much noise as you want to, listen to music, and help yourself to the food or drink of your choice. You have complete bodily freedom, and you can give birth either on your own bed or on the floor. You can be alone, or share the experience with people of your own choosing.

After the birth, you and your family can all be together to enjoy the special time of celebration. You can sleep when your baby sleeps and have your baby with you in bed, day or night. It is usually easier to establish breastfeeding and to learn to care for your baby in these conditions.

For a home birth, you are expected to fall into the "low-risk" category, medically speaking. That is, you should be in good health with no problems in your pregnancy and no history of illness or obstetric complications that could affect the birth. Sometimes, however, a mother who is "high-risk" may also be better off staying at home, where she is assured of the careful attention of a skilled attendant.

When planning a home birth, be sure to arrange suitable backup care in case complications arise and you need to be transferred to the hospital.

The Birth Room

> "I went upstairs to the bedroom that I had prepared for the birth. There was a foam mattress in front of the fire, covered with a clean sheet; an enormous beanbag chair, also covered with a sheet, resting against the foot of my bed; and a small stool to sit on between contractions."

Arrange a pleasant environment where you have several alternatives for changing positions. No special equipment is needed—you probably already have everything you'll want. Make sure you have a good supply of cushions and a low stool or pile of big, heavy books for supporting you in a squatting position. Extra heating should be available, as the baby will need to be kept very warm immediately after the birth. Dim light is most conducive for relaxation in labor, but one lamp should be handy for the midwife or doctor in case it is needed. Your midwife or doctor will provide you with a list of supplies needed for the delivery; keep them in a box or drawer in the birth room.

It is quite likely that you will give birth not in your prepared room but in another place entirely. It is not uncommon for babies to be born in the bathroom, where the mother has a feeling of privacy and is near to water. Unless your labor is very short, you will want to make use of the bathtub or shower. It is unlikely that your baby will be born in the water; however, this is perfectly safe if this does happen, and it may be very enjoyable. It is usually best to wait until you are halfway through your labor (about 5 centimeters dilation) before spending long periods in the bath—warm water is most helpful if you use it only after you've begun to really need it (see chapter 8).

> *"I decided to relax in a bath. On feeling a contraction I stepped out of it to lean against the sink and to slowly rotate my body as if spinning a Hula-Hoop. I continued in this way, topping up the bath with hot water until I had three consecutive contractions each lasting about a minute."*

After the Birth

After the birth it is not necessary to dress the baby. In fact, it's wonderful to be naked together, and the skin-to-skin contact enhances bonding. Your baby will be more comfortable, too, loosely wrapped and close to your body. Have plenty of soft towels or receiving blankets handy (small, soft flannel sheets are fine), as the baby needs to be kept warm. For the first day or two after the birth (or longer), it is best for the baby to be close to the warmth of your body and the familiar sound of your heartbeat. It is ideal for you to sleep together (and to bathe together) at this time. Sleeping together will ensure that the baby gets every opportunity to nurse and thereby takes in plenty of the valuable colostrum, which contains antibodies to strengthen his or her immunity to infection. Because colostrum also has a laxative effect, it prepares the digestive tract to absorb the milk that will probably "come in" on the second or third day after the birth.

In the hours after the birth, your midwife will help to clean up, and then she will leave. It's worth thinking in advance of what you will need at this time and having it all handy near your bedside. You will need a bowl for warm water and cloths to clean the baby after the first bowel movement occurs. (The first excrement is a dark green or black sticky substance called meconium. In a day or so the excrement will become yellowish.) You will need diapers of some sort, too. A diaper service, which can provide special small diapers for newborns, makes life easier in the first weeks. You will use about a dozen diapers a day! A waterproof mattress pad will prevent stains on your mattress, and a night-light, water carafe, and telephone are all handy to have in the bedroom. It is also a good idea to have some almond oil or calendula cream to put on your nipples after the baby sucks, to help prevent soreness (see chapter 8).

You will probably feel marvelous after the birth, but take care to get enough rest and sleep, and to use your energy for nursing and taking care of your baby. Unless you plan for some private time each day, you could find yourself entertaining visitors all day after a home birth. You need plenty of time to get to know your new baby quietly.

ACTIVE BIRTH IN THE HOSPITAL

There is no reason why active birth cannot be put into practice in any environment suitable for birth. If you are having your baby in the hospital, find out beforehand whether the staff will allow you to move around and use upright positions for delivery. Take a tour of the hospital maternity area, and ask questions about everything you want to know. Find out if the hospital provides the following items:

- A low stool or birthstool, useful for supporting you in the squatting position;
- Extra bed pillows;
- A cotton blanket that can be wrapped in a pillow case for kneeling on;
- A beanbag chair; and
- A tape recorder.

Note the whereabouts of showers or bathtubs so you can use them during labor.

Explore the possibilities of the bed. Most delivery beds are adjustable: the bed can be raised or lowered, the backrest and foot can be raised or lowered independently, and sometimes the foot and its mattress can be removed altogether. This mattress serves well as a cushion to lean on. Many beds also have squatting bars.

You may want to ask—

- Is it possible to give birth on the floor rather than on a bed or delivery table?
- Does the staff have hand-held fetal heart monitors (Doptones) that can be used easily when I am in an upright position, without disturbing the flow of labor?

You may want to learn more about the hospital by taking its childbirth preparation class, even if you will be taking a private class as well. But take care to resist any pressure to fall in line with hospital routines.

More hospitals are recognizing the advantages of activity during labor and upright positions for birth, although many still emphasize intervention and the use of technology. It is important for you to find out the hospital's policies and routines well in advance, and it is your right to change to a hospital that suits your needs. Changing hospitals, of course, may mean changing birth attendants. You can ask the hospital of your choice for names of doctors and midwives who attend births there.

> *"I had previously stated that I wanted no enema, monitor, drugs, or cuts unless absolutely necessary, and once the midwife confirmed my wishes, no more was said."*

What to Take with You

When you go to the hospital in labor, take a large, firm cushion or two (measuring roughly three feet square) or a beanbag chair to lean on, if the hospital provides neither. The cushion should be firm, as thick as possible, and, of course, very clean. You will need several bed pillows as well; bring some if the hospital doesn't provide extras.

Bring a stool if the hospital doesn't provide one. It is also a good idea to take a pad for kneeling on. A firm cotton or synthetic pillow, or a piece of foam rubber two inches thick in a clean pillow case is ideal. You can use it on the floor or on the bed to protect your knees.

Many couples like to take a tape recorder, if the hospital doesn't provide one, along with the music of their choice. This is often delightfully relaxing for the attendants as well as the mother.

Take your own nightgown to wear, as you will want to look and feel good. A short cotton one that can open in front (or a man's shirt or pajama top) is convenient for nursing and easy to take off. Also bring socks in case the room is chilly.

You might bring a sponge (natural, if possible) for refreshing yourself in labor and, later, bathing the baby.

You may like to take your own herbal tea bags and a jar of honey. A spoonful every now and then in herbal tea will ensure that your blood-sugar level doesn't drop, and will eliminate the need for an intravenous glucose drip. Apple juice or red grape juice will have the same effect, as will glucose tablets (don't take citrus juice—it's too acidic).

Of course, your partner will need some food and some coins for the pay phone, if necessary.

Movements for Labor

Stay at home for the early part of the first stage. After you are admitted to the hospital, you will be examined to see how far you have dilated. The position and well-being of the baby will be checked. Some hospitals offer enemas, but you can refuse if you would rather not have one, as it is not necessary. When you arrive in the hospital, don't be surprised if things slow down for a while. As soon as you relax and settle down, the rhythm of the labor will pick up.

A shower or bath is very relaxing. Enjoy it! If you have a long first stage, you may enjoy using the shower from time to time. You can walk around the labor room or up and down the corridor. When labor gets stronger, you may like to stand at the side of the bed, place your big cushion in front of you, and lean forward onto the cushion during contractions, with one foot on the stool. Another good idea is to sit on a chair facing the bed and lean forward onto the cushion.

You can use the stool to support you in a squatting position—place a pillow on it, or ask the nurse or midwife for a disposable paper pad. Or squat on the floor, holding on to the bar of the bed for support.

When labor gets very strong, you can get up on the delivery bed if you are expected or want to do so. Lift up the backrest, and pile your cushions against it so you can lean forward onto them to rest between contractions, completely supported in the kneeling position.

You can also squat holding on to the backrest. Alternatively, your partner can support you while standing behind the bed—pull it out from the wall a little—or at the side. Try squatting sideways on the bed, putting your arms around your partner's shoulders for support. You can squat facing away from your partner, while he or she supports you from behind, or you can squat leaning forward onto your pile of cushions. Or use the squatting bar, if one is available. Follow your instincts, and adapt the environment to suit your needs.

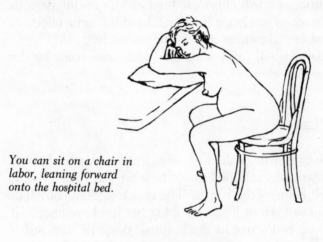

You can sit on a chair in labor, leaning forward onto the hospital bed.

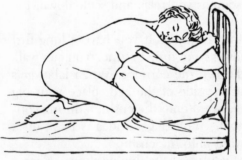

Or kneel on the bed.

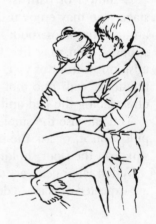

Or squat on the bed while your partner supports you.

The Second Stage in the Hospital

If you are able to remain on the floor, you can follow the advice given in chapter 6 for the second stage. Some hospitals are willing to place a mattress on the floor for women who wish to squat, but others still insist that the second stage take place on a bed. The kneeling position presents no problem on a bed; simply kneel forward onto a pile of cushions. In case you wish to squat on the bed, these are the ways of being supported:

Squatting with Two Supporters

Squat on the bed with a pillow under your heels. Your supporters should stand at your sides on either side of the bed. If they are more or less the same height, you will probably be able to put one arm around each of their shoulders quite comfortably. They can each put one arm around

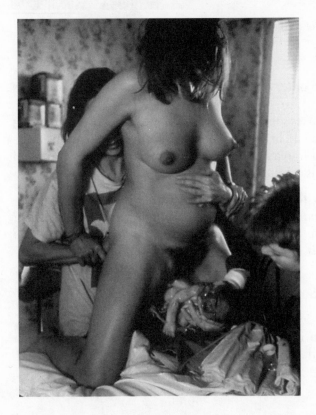

As the mother kneels upright, the baby is born on the hospital bed.

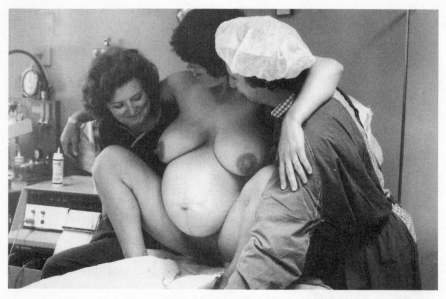

Partners stand at the side of the bed and support the mother in the squatting position.

your back and use the other arm to support you under each knee, if this is comfortable for you.

If the second stage takes some time, wait until the baby's head is coming to go into a squat, to avoid becoming too tired. For variation and resting, you can come forward into a kneeling position. It is also possible to stand up during contractions, by holding on to your supporters' shoulders.

> "I was helped by the doctor and my husband into a squatting posi-
> tion. This was marvelous! I could push so much more easily, and it
> was a comfort to feel their strength helping support me. I stayed
> squatting, as this brought her head down very quickly!"

Squatting with One Supporter

Another way of being supported in the squatting position is from behind. This works well when it is possible to lower the backrest. Your partner stands behind the bed and supports you as in the "standing" squat in chapter 6.

This can also be done (perhaps more comfortably for both of you) with you squatting sideways on the bed, if the midwife is willing to assist from the other side of the bed.

Another possibility is for your partner to sit behind you on the pile of cushions or beanbag chair on the bed. You squat between your partner's legs, using his or her body for support.

Squatting with a Squatting Bar

Lastly, some delivery beds are equipped with a detachable bar that can quickly be inserted into openings in the sides of the bedframe. You can hold on to the bar for stability and support.

These examples are all drawn from situations where people have managed to find their own ways of making use of whatever is available and acceptable to the hospital. It is important to visit the hospital during pregnancy to get an idea of the possibilities and to discuss them with the staff. If an upright position turns out to be tiring or uncomfortable, try the side-lying position in preference to semireclining.

Your partner can stand behind you to support you as you give birth squatting on the bed.

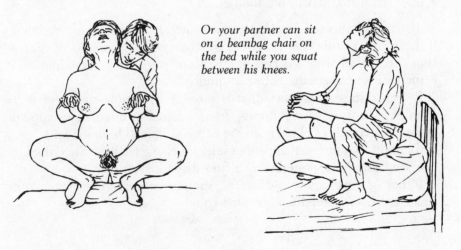

Or your partner can sit on a beanbag chair on the bed while you squat between his knees.

FETAL DISTRESS

This happens when a baby is not getting enough oxygen. There are usually two symptoms:

1. The baby's heart rate falls or rises until it is consistently slower or faster than the normal limits of 120 to 160 beats per minute.
2. The baby's anal sphincter relaxes, passing some of the first fecal matter (meconium) into the amniotic fluid, and turning it brown or green. This can lead to a secondary complication: if the baby inhales amniotic fluid, the meconium can congest the lungs and cause respiration problems.

When both meconium staining and an abnormal heart rate are present, the baby is very likely in trouble.

Fetal distress may be caused by—

- compression of the mother's major internal blood vessels, as in the reclining position;
- prolonged labor;
- premature induction;
- large doses of analgesic medication, such as Demerol;
- placental dysfunction;
- prolapse, entanglement, or compression of the umbilical cord; or
- diabetes or toxemia in the mother.

To avoid or alleviate fetal distress, keep active and upright during labor. If the baby's heartbeat is irregular, try changing positions to vertical or kneeling. If fetal distress occurs in the second stage, then a standing squat is the best way to get the baby out quickly.

If fetal distress is suspected, it is possible to double-check for it by changing the form of monitoring (from external to internal, usually) or by taking a sample of blood from the baby's scalp and testing it for oxygen and carbon dioxide levels and other relevant characteristics. Such double-checking should be done before a firm diagnosis is made.

It may be necessary to use forceps, vacuum extraction, episiotomy, or cesarean section to help a distressed baby.

MONITORING THE BABY FOR ACTIVE BIRTH

Your baby's heartbeat will be checked regularly during labor, every hour or so. If labor is progressing well, the nurse or midwife may not need to check it as often and may rely on her intuition. In the second stage the fetal heart may be checked more frequently, but, again, this may not be necessary.

The ordinary stethoscope is perfectly adequate for checking the fetal heart. The nurse or midwife may ask you to sit up vertically or lean back slightly while she checks the heartbeat. Some enterprising midwives manage to use a stethoscope from underneath while the woman in labor is on all fours. The stethoscope may actually be easier to use in this position.

The most common type of fetal heart monitor is the hand-held ultrasound monitor, which magnifies the sound of the baby's heartbeat. These are relatively inexpensive, so most hospitals and doctors have them. They can be used with the woman in any upright position, and they cause no discomfort to the mother, or, apparently, to the baby (although the effects on the baby have not yet been adequately researched).

The abdominal belt monitors most commonly used in hospitals present certain problems. The mother must wear two belts strapped around her abdomen—one to measure the contractions and one the baby's heartbeat—which generally confines her to the semireclining position. Many women complain that the belts are very uncomfortable. The contractions are certainly more painful in the semireclining position, and there is a real contradiction here: the monitors are used to detect fetal distress while confining the mother to the position most likely to induce it! Also, we know that machines often break down or don't work properly, and when attendants rely solely on machinery to detect distress, they may ignore their instincts. As a compromise to continuous monitoring, some hospitals ask that you have the belt monitor attached for twenty minutes to obtain a continuous reading. This is usually unnecessary, and it may be disturbing if you find the belts uncomfortable, although some women do not object. Women from my classes have successfully used belt monitors in the kneeling position, which eliminates some of the problems.

"I had to get onto the delivery bed and be monitored, as the doctor was worried because the baby was small. As soon as I lay down on the bed the contractions became painful, and so as soon as the monitors were attached I turned over and knelt up on the bed. Immediately the pain disappeared and I could cope well with the contractions."

The other form of monitoring that may be used, often in addition to the belt monitor, is the scalp electrode monitor. Designed for use on babies who are at risk, this was never intended to be routinely used for normal labor. The electrode is attached by a tiny spiral wire or hook through the cervix to the baby's scalp. This form of monitoring allows the mother some mobility, depending on the length of the cord and the flexibility of the attendants. However, the disadvantage here is that the membranes have to be ruptured in order to attach the electrode, and this has its attendant risks—it accelerates labor, sometimes violently, and increases the risk of infection. Rupturing the membranes also causes unnecessary pressure from the contracting uterus on the infant's head (see "Inducing or Accelerating Labor"). The effect of attaching the electrode to the baby, as a first touch from the outside world, is also questionable. Some babies are left with a small wound on the head and occasionally a permanent tiny bald patch where the electrode was attached.

In the event of a threatened complication, such as when the attendant detects a persistently irregular heartbeat, scalp electrode monitoring may be appropriate, as it is considered to be more accurate than a belt monitor, and in such a case the baby's safety is a priority. But several studies show that routine electronic fetal monitoring—by the external or the internal method—offers no advantage to mothers or babies over listening with a hand-held stethoscope. In fact, when electronic fetal monitoring becomes routine, the cesarean rate usually rises.[1]

A radio-operated (telemetry) monitor allows the mother complete mobility, although it may necessitate rupturing the membranes to attach a scalp electrode. If electronic monitoring is necessary, ask if a telemetry unit is available.

In normal labor, monitoring should not interfere with the normal physiology. As soon as it does, the monitor itself can become the cause of the problems it is intended to prevent.

EATING IN LABOR

When you are in labor your stomach and bowels will want to empty themselves of their contents. It is not a good idea, therefore, to eat large meals or foods that are hard to digest. But if you have a long labor, you are going to need some food to sustain you, or you may become exhausted. If this happens, you will feel tired and weak, and labor can cease to progress well. Medically, this state is known as *ketosis*. It is diagnosed when your urine is tested and found to contain acetone. If your body is short of glucose it will burn other fuel in the body, such as fat. Acetone in your urine and ketones in your blood are the acidic products of fat metabolism.

Most hospitals do not allow a woman in labor to eat anything at all (in case you need a cesarean with general anesthesia). To prevent ketosis, they prefer to attach an intravenous glucose drip. This usually means you are restricted to the reclining position, and you may also feel hungry!

Ketosis can be avoided by the following:

- At home in early labor, eat a light meal, such as a slice of toast, an egg, yogurt with wheat germ and honey, or some soup.
- If you are hungry during a long labor, eat another light, breakfasty snack, or a few spoonfuls of light, nourishing soup might be enjoyable.
- Have some form of sugar every now and then, such as a spoonful of honey in boiling water or herb tea, or some red grape or apple juice. If you do become slightly ketotic, take some glucose tablets, and sip non-citrus fruit juice between every contraction. Once you are in strong labor, sips of water are all you will need or want.

INTERNAL EXAMINATIONS

These are done by the nurse or midwife to assess the progress of the labor. She inserts her fingers into your vagina and feels the cervix and the top of the baby's head to gather information about the dilation and the presentation of the baby.

When a woman is active in labor and labor is obviously progressing well, it is not necessary to make these examinations often, and sometimes they are not needed at all. Most attendants like to examine internally at the end of the first stage to check if dilation is complete. Some, however, prefer to rely on other signs, such as the mother's desire to grasp something or get down onto the floor in the all-fours position, a "bearing-down" sound in her voice, a bulging of the perineal tissues, and dilation of the anus. These attendants avoid disturbing the onset of the expulsive reflex, and do an internal exam only if there is doubt that things are progressing normally.

You yourself may wish to be examined to know how far you have dilated. Some women, however, complain that it is uncomfortable to be touched in this most tender part during labor. Internal examinations can be done, very gently, between rather than during contractions, and in a position most comfortable to you. It is possible for an attendant to examine a woman standing up (with one leg up on a chair), sitting on the edge of a chair, or on all fours. Any of these positions may be far less uncomfortable than the semireclining position.

Most nurses and midwives have been trained to examine women in a semireclining position, and many, understandably, do not like to change their ways. Perhaps you could ask to try another position first, agreeing to lie back if your attendant has any difficulty; he or she will probably discover that it is just as easy to examine you upright. If, for some reason, the attendant requires you to lie back, you can get up again when she has finished. Breathing deeply and relaxing as much as possible while being examined should help.

The all-fours position offers the attendant an excellent view of what is happening as the baby is born. In fact, as far as view and access go, this position is ideal. The problem here is that the attendant's routine is literally turned upside down—but this should present little difficulty once the decision is made to try something new. When attending a birth in which the woman follows her own instincts, the midwife or doctor is also, by necessity, more spontaneous and more instinctive. In the few places in the Western world where birth is normally managed in a spontaneous rather than routine way, the outcomes tend to be much better than those in our high-tech hospitals (see chapter 1).

If you are in a squatting position for birth, the midwife or doctor will need to rely on his or her hands to feel the baby's progress, or else bend down to look. As the pelvis is more open and perineum more relaxed in this position, there is less need for examination and rarely any need to guard the perineum.

After the baby's head emerges, the midwife or doctor will check with a finger to see if the umbilical cord is around the baby's neck. This is a common occurrence, and all the attendant normally has to do is to loosen the cord by pulling it a little, and to slip it over the baby's head and body as the baby emerges, or just after. Midwives experienced with the squatting position tell us that a cord around the neck presents no problems and can be handled in exactly the same way as if the mother were reclining.

In the rare case of the cord being wound twice or more times around the neck, it is safest for the mother to be squatting (preferably in a standing squat), so the pelvis is wide open and the baby can be born much quicker than if the mother were reclining. She should sit down as soon as the baby is born so the doctor or midwife can more easily unravel the cord. Cutting the cord is not desirable in this situation, unless it is preventing the baby from coming out, in which case a supported standing squat or a kneeling position is imperative for safety. Once the child is born, the cord is usually quickly unraveled. It is left to stop pulsating while the baby is placed between the mother's legs on his or her belly.

INDUCING OR ACCELERATING LABOR

Labor usually happens naturally when the time is right. But sometimes the doctor may recommend starting it artificially, with an induction, and sometimes a slow labor may be artificially speeded up.

Labor may be induced because a medical problem, such as preeclampsia or diabetes, makes continuing the pregnancy dangerous for the mother or the baby. Some doctors want to induce labor when the bag of waters has been broken for a long time (12 to 24 hours) and contractions have failed to start spontaneously, in which case the risk of infection is increased. Often labor is induced because the mother has passed her due date by two weeks or more without beginning labor. The concern here is that the placenta may not function well after 40 weeks, so the baby could be malnourished. But since pregnancies normally vary in length, being late according to the calendar is not alone a good reason for induction. If the mother and baby are carefully observed and no signs of complication arise, there is no harm in waiting for labor to start on its own.

When labor must start, you may be able to induce it yourself. Lovemaking is a pleasant way to do this. The prostaglandin in semen softens the cervix, and the relaxation and orgasm may start you off. Nipple stimulation can also bring on labor. Exercise may stimulate labor contractions, and so may bowel stimulation through an enema or a dose of castor oil taken orally (consult your doctor or midwife for guidelines). Both enemas and castor oil may cause cramping and diarrhea, however.

I find that a very successful way to bring on labor is through acupuncture. If labor does not start within 24 hours after an acupuncture treatment, your midwife or doctor may be able to help by gently massaging the cervix. This stimulates the production of prostaglandins by the tiny glands in the cervix. (This should not be done after the membranes have ruptured, as it would increase the risk of infection.)

If none of these measures work, prostaglandin gel can be placed within or on the outside of the cervix to soften it. This treatment may start contractions, too. Although long used in Europe, prostaglandin gel has not been approved by the Food and Drug Administration, so it is not available in all hospitals, and its formula varies. Since its possible side effects include rapid blood pressure changes, nausea, and unusually strong contractions, it should be used with caution.

If labor has started but is very slow, there is usually no cause for concern provided the baby's heartbeat is normal, the mother is coping and feeling well, and the cervix is dilating. Many women take a long time sinking into the first stage, and others need time to let the baby descend to be born in the second stage. Sometimes hunger can cause delay. Perhaps the mother is afraid of something she cannot express, or is struggling inwardly with inhibitions. If she is given understanding, time, and privacy, she will probably find her own way of overcoming her difficulties.

It is quite normal for some labors to stop and start during the first stage. It often happens that labor is very slow at first but suddenly advances rapidly. A woman can take 12 hours or more going from 0 to 6 centimeters, and 10 minutes from 6 centimeters to full dilation.

Generally, the best way to help a slow labor is to darken the room and leave the mother alone for a while. Immersion in water is often very helpful after 5 centimeters dilation. Walking, perhaps outdoors if the weather permits, can help (stop to lean forward during contractions).

The more vertical postures will accelerate labor by helping the baby to descend and exerting more pressure on the cervix. Squatting is likely to intensify the contractions. Movement will probably accelerate the labor, and half-kneeling, half-squatting can speed up dilation of the cervix.

The hospital's usual means of inducing or accelerating labor are, first, an oxytocin (Pitocin) intravenous drip and, second, artificial rupture of the membranes. Pitocin causes contractions that are stronger and closer together than those of normal labor. Often having two peaks, these contractions are certainly more difficult to cope with than normal ones. When the contractions are very powerful, they can interrupt the blood flow to the placenta, which increases the likelihood of fetal distress. Careful fetal monitoring is mandatory during administration of Pitocin.

Fortunately, some hospitals have mobile intravenous drips that enable you to stand or walk while receiving Pitocin. The fetal heart monitor can also be worn while you are upright. You need a good pile of cushions or a beanbag chair to support your body in the kneeling position so you can rest between contractions.

Artificial rupture of the membranes is done by inserting an instrument like a crochet hook through the cervix, and breaking the membranes that surround the baby. The amniotic fluid then begins to drain, and contractions usually intensify. In some hospitals this is a routine procedure on admission.

The disadvantages of rupturing the membranes are—

- The protective fluid between the baby's head and the contracting uterus is lost, so there is more pressure on the head and on the cord from the powerful uterine contractions. This can cause a decrease in the flow of blood to and from the baby, and some evidence indicates that the baby's heart rate slows slightly.
- There is increased risk of infection for the mother once the membranes are ruptured.
- As with Pitocin, contractions can suddenly become much stronger and more painful after the membranes are ruptured. It can be very difficult to cope with this rapid increase in intensity.
- The baby is probably more comfortable with water between its body and the powerfully contracting uterus.

The painful contractions caused by induction may lead a woman to accept a pain reliever or anesthesia, which can weaken her contractions and lessen her ability to push. The result is often a cesarean section. When artificial rupture of the membranes fails to induce labor, the risk of infection in the mother is increased, and, again, the final result may be a cesarean section.

Inducing labor on the basis of dates alone also threatens the health of the baby. Whether by Pitocin or artificial rupture of the membranes, induction increases the likelihood of the baby being born premature, in need of special care away from his or her mother, and at risk for infection, breathing difficulties, and severe jaundice.

But if labor is not progressing after a long time has elapsed (12 to 24 hours) and there does not seem to be an obvious reason, one should allow for the possibility that there may be some physical problem, such as the presentation of the baby or the internal shape of the mother's pelvis, and help may be needed.

SLOWING DOWN LABOR

If labor is progressing very fast, the all-fours position can prevent the mother from feeling overwhelmed. The knee-chest position may help to slow down the contractions (see page 131). Very slow deep breathing can also be helpful.

UNUSUAL PRESENTATIONS

Before the birth, the baby usually lies with its head engaged in the pelvis in what is known as the anterior position: the baby's back lies against the mother's abdominal wall, and the limbs are folded in front, facing the mother's spine. The head is flexed well forward, ready for birth. In this position the baby's descent through the birth canal is easiest. However, sometimes there are variations in the way the baby lies.

With the use of upright positions for labor and birth, these variations can usually be managed without intervention. When the mother moves about in labor, the baby is more likely to be able to move into the anterior position, and her movements will also help the baby descend.

Posterior Position

This position is fairly common. It may be caused by the position of the placenta; babies usually face their placentas *in utero*, so if the placenta is on the front wall of the uterus, the baby may be lying posterior. In the posterior position, the baby lies with its spine against the mother's spine and its limbs towards the mother's abdominal wall. Usually a baby will rotate into the anterior position just before or during labor, but sometimes a baby remains posterior for the birth. With the use of upright positions, this doesn't usually present any serious problems; however, there is more pressure from the baby's head on the mother's sacrum, which usually results in painful "back labor." Also, since the fit between the baby's head and the pelvis isn't quite as good, and the head may be slowly rotating into the anterior position, the labor is often slower.

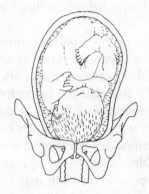 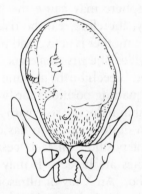

A baby in posterior position   *A baby in anterior position*

The best way to deal with a posterior presentation is to kneel, leaning forward over cushions or a beanbag chair, so the weight of the baby is taken off your back, thus easing the pain. When you are in this position, the heaviest part of the baby—the spine and the back of the head—will tend to gravitate downwards, and this will encourage the baby to rotate into the anterior position.

Rotating your hips in this position will help the baby to descend. Rotating the hips while standing up and leaning forward is also useful.

For the second stage, a full or standing squat is usually best, as it allows maximum opening of the pelvis and help from gravity. Sometimes kneeling is most comfortable for the delivery, and it may be most practical, as the mother need not change position and the baby can rotate as it comes out.

Breech Presentation

When a baby is lying in a breech presentation, its head is uppermost and its bottom or legs are presenting first. It is quite possible for a baby to be born vaginally in this position, but there are ways of gently encouraging a breech baby to turn before labor starts. It is desirable to try these methods, as a breech birth may be problematic in that the head of the baby is the largest part of its body and will be emerging last. If the umbilical cord, emerging before the head, becomes compressed, the blood supply to the baby may be affected. Also, the stimulation of the baby's skin by the atmosphere may cause the baby to breathe before the head is out. Any delay, therefore, can be risky.

When a mother is active and upright in labor, the risks are minimized, and, provided the first stage goes well and a supported standing squat is used, most breech births are uncomplicated. Practitioners who often use upright squatting positions for breech births find that the help of gravity is essential in reducing risks with a breech presentation. It may be difficult to find an obstetrician who has experience with vaginal breech birth in an upright position; in fact, cesarean sections are performed routinely when babies are breech. It may be possible, however, to arrange for a trial of labor. An X ray or ultrasound scan prior to the birth may reassure both mother and obstetrician that the baby will be able to pass through the pelvis in a breech position.

Most babies lying breech will turn of their own accord before the birth. This may happen just before labor starts. Walking for an hour a day in the open air will encourage the baby to turn. Since the head is the heaviest

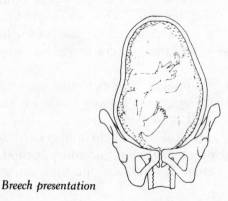

Breech presentation

part of the baby's body, it will tend to move down with gravity when encouraged by the walking motion.

If your baby is breech at 35 weeks, stop squatting, to prevent the baby's buttocks from engaging in the pelvic brim. Try the following exercise, discussing it first with your doctor or midwife. (A word of caution: a lot of babies who are lying breech turn spontaneously six weeks before birth, so don't do anything until five weeks before the due date—that is, 35 weeks). Ask your doctor or midwife to help you to feel how your baby is lying before you start. Together, try to discover the exact location of the head, the limbs, the baby's spine, and the placenta. A breech position can be confirmed by an ultrasound scan.

Exercise to Encourage a Breech Baby to Turn

(Caution: If you find that you are dizzy lying on your back, then you should not do this exercise. Try to spend time in the knee-chest position instead; see page 131.)

1. Place a large, firm cushion or two on the floor, and lie on your back with your hips raised up on the cushion and your head on the floor, so that your pelvis is higher than your head. You can place a pillow under your head if you feel breathless. In this position the baby will drop slightly away from the pelvis and may begin to move. Relax and breathe deeply.

2. Using a vegetable oil, massage your belly with your hands to gently encourage your baby to turn. Ask your midwife or doctor beforehand which would be the easiest way for the baby to turn, and massage in that direction only. Use gentle but firm and consistent pressure.

Do this exercise for 10 minutes at a time, several times throughout the day.

It will probably take at least a week or two before the baby turns. When

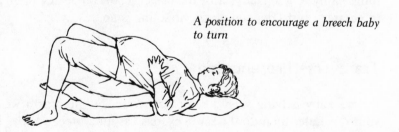

A position to encourage a breech baby to turn

it happens, you will probably feel the change. Arrange beforehand with your doctor or midwife to have an examination as soon as you suspect that the baby has turned. If the exam confirms that the head is down, then stop doing the exercise and start squatting to help the head to engage.

If the exercise and walks alone don't do the trick, you may want to use homoeopathy and acupuncture in combination with them. A physician or midwife who practices homeopathy may prescribe the homeopathic remedy pulsatilla (10m). A single dose of this remedy may stimulate a baby to move, as may a simple acupuncturist's treatment called *moksha*, in which heat (rather than a needle) is applied to a point on the little toe. This can be done while you are lying in the position just described. If your partner accompanies you to the session, the acupuncturist can teach you to continue the treatment at home.

After all these efforts a baby will usually turn. But if your baby is still breech in labor, and if your obstetrician is agreeable, stay vertical and use the standing squat to bear down. This will give your baby as much room as possible and maximum help from gravity.

If the baby needs help in the second stage, forceps are usually used. Michel Odent often stresses that the supported standing squat is imperative for a breech delivery without forceps, as it allows for the rapid and most efficient descent of the baby through the pelvis. Odent believes that this method of delivering a breech is safer than a forceps delivery, in which there is always a risk of damage to the baby from the forceps. With the standing squat, episiotomy is rarely needed. Occasionally, to speed up delivery of the head, an episiotomy is done (while the mother remains standing) just before the baby's head emerges (see "Episiotomy").

If the first stage does not progress satisfactorily, the baby must be born by cesarean section. However, it is generally not necessary to do a cesarean until there has been a trial of labor. In fact, it is usually better to wait until the mother goes into labor spontaneously, so it is certain that the baby is ready to be born and will be capable of breathing through the lungs easily. Once labor starts, the obstetrician can decide upon a vaginal or cesarean birth depending on how things go.

Transverse Presentation

If your baby is lying sideways, or transverse, by the fourth week before your due date, then do the same exercise as for a breech baby. Kneeling

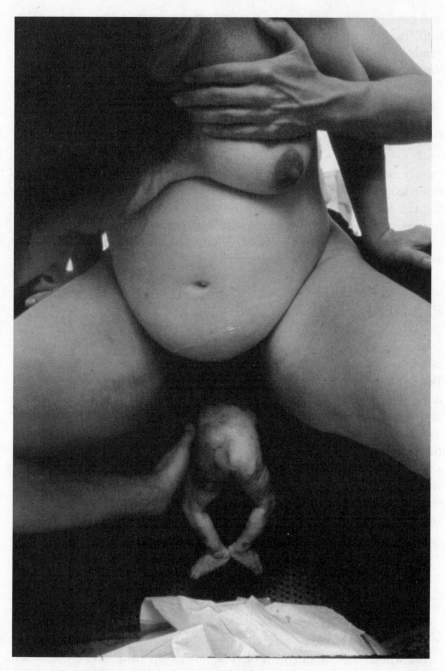

A supported upright squat maximizes the help of gravity when a baby is breech at birth.

and rotating your hips during the first stage may help to get your baby into the correct position. If the baby remains transverse or breech, a cesarean section is necessary, but the baby may well turn head down at the very last minute. It's worth a try! Walking for an hour every day may help the baby's head to descend.

Extended Neck

In very rare instances, a baby's head is at an unusual angle, with the neck extended rather than flexed. This can prevent the head from passing through the pelvis. If you are moving your body intuitively during labor, however, the head may settle into the right position, and a normal birth can follow. If the neck remains extended, vacuum extraction, forceps, or a cesarean section may be necessary.

PERINEAL TEARS

In the second stage of labor, as the baby's head comes down to the base of the pelvis and crowns, the perineal tissues soften and stretch open. When the mother is in the squatting or kneeling position, the pelvis opens to its widest. The back or sacral part of the pelvic floor draws backwards and relaxes, allowing maximum opening of the vagina. In this position a tear is less likely than if the mother is semireclining, since pressure from the descending head is exerted evenly around the vagina. (When the mother is semireclining, the pressure comes directly on the perineum, which cannot stretch as effectively in this position.) However, tears are a natural hazard of birth. They usually heal without difficulty, and the stitching to repair them is done with a local anesthetic (see chapter 6).

How to Avoid A Tear

- During pregnancy, practice the yoga-based exercises and pelvic floor exercises regularly.
- In the last six weeks of pregnancy, you can massage the perineum and the whole vaginal area with olive oil after your bath. Some midwives recommend stretching the perineum with your fingers. These are tradi-

tional practices in many cultures, but your perineum will soften naturally anyway.

- Give birth in a darkened room or other place where you feel safe and private, with as few people present as possible, so you can let go without feeling watched.
- Use upright squatting or kneeling positions for the birth of the baby.
- Don't rush, hold your breath for long periods, or push too forcefully in the second stage. Holding your breath for long periods tenses your pelvic floor and can affect your baby's oxygen supply. Let your uterus be your guide; follow your own urges to deliver your child. If you don't try to hurry the process, your perineum should have time to stretch.
- Ask the midwife or nurse not to swab you down with disinfectant, as this simply washes away the natural lubrication and will make a tear more likely.
- In natural positions it is generally not necessary for the midwife or doctor to guard the perineum. However, if the tissues seem very tight, it is very helpful for the attendant to apply hot compresses. A small towel, diaper, or washcloth can be used. Your partner or attendant should pour almost boiling water over several of them in a basin. As soon as they are touchable, he or she should wring one out and fold it, test it on the wrist to be sure it is warm but not burning, and place it on the perineum. A new one should be used after each contraction. This is very soothing, and it helps to bring blood to the area and relax the tissues. A quick and easy compress can be made by using a sanitary towel and hot water from the tap. The attendant just squeezes out excess water, and applies the compress.
- Use your own hands to feel the baby's head when it begins to crown and to ease the tissues or even massage them with a little oil. According to Dr. Michael Rosenthal, founder of the Family Birthing Center in Upland, California, mothers who use their own hands to help the baby out rarely tear.
- Feel free to shout spontaneously as you push and as the baby emerges— as your throat releases, so will your perineum!

EPISIOTOMY

An episiotomy is a surgical incision or cut that is made in the perineum with scissors to enlarge the vaginal opening. A local anesthetic is injected into the area beforehand, so the incision is painless, although there is usually some discomfort afterwards, while it is healing. The cut is roughly ½ to 1 inch long and is made through the skin and muscle of the perineum, either down the midline or at an angle. (A natural tear is more superficial and usually does not go through the muscle layer.) The cut is sewn up after the birth.

In a report on episiotomy published by the National Childbirth Trust of Britain in 1981, Dr. M. J. House wrote, "We obstetricians teach that episiotomy prevents tears and reduces the likelihood of prolapse in the future—but we have little or no evidence for making these statements. Not only is there no evidence that episiotomy prevents tears but there is some evidence to the contrary."[2] The authors of the report found that generally episiotomy is unnecessary, and that a natural tear heals better and presents fewer physical and psychological problems than a cut. In my work I have exactly the same findings.

Although many professionals now recognize that episiotomy is performed unnecessarily, it has become a routine procedure in almost every hospital in the United States. The most common obstetric intervention, episiotomy is often performed without the consent of the mother, who may not need it at all.

When a woman is active in labor, when upright positions are used for the second stage, and when the mother is encouraged to take her time and follow her own instincts, rather than to push forcefully, episiotomy is seldom needed. When the perineum is tight, warm compresses can help bring blood to the tissues so they can stretch more easily, making episiotomy often avoidable. It is only in rare situations, when the perineum is especially tight, or when an episiotomy can save the baby's life by speeding up the delivery, that this intervention is really necessary. When birth is active, episiotomy can take its rightful place as an emergency procedure.

When an episiotomy is required, the all-fours position may be the best posture to use. With it the baby receives a better supply of oxygen, as there is no pressure on the internal blood vessels; the mother is more comfortable; the perineal tissues are most accessible to the attendant and relaxed; and extended tearing is less likely, as there is less pressure on the perineum when the baby's head emerges. Also, if the baby is distressed, the greater opening of the pelvic outlet in this position helps to speed up the delivery.

If you have an episiotomy, the stitching should be done soon after the birth to prevent blood loss and infection and to promote healing. Local anesthetic is essential.

As the aftereffects of episiotomy can be very painful, and the actual operation, though brief, can interrupt one of the most intimate and deeply personal experiences of your life, it is well worth discussing this subject with your attendants before the event and putting your wishes in writing.

EPIDURAL ANESTHESIA

Activity and upright positions in labor increase your chances of giving birth naturally. But if an epidural becomes necessary, you can benefit by using gravity-effective positions along with the anesthesia.

When you are given an epidural, side-lying is preferable to semireclining during the first stage, but change sides from time to time. You can sit upright and lean forward slightly or sit on the edge of the bed and lean forward with the attendant's assistance. Changing positions is extremely beneficial, as epidurals often cause loss of muscle power and therefore less efficient contractions; movement counteracts this effect. The reclining position may also reduce blood flow to the uterus, so side-lying will help to prevent fetal distress.

For delivery, side-lying is preferable to lying back. If the epidural has worn off, you may be able to manage supported squatting or kneeling.

At the Garden Hospital in London, most women who have epidurals squat, with help, to give birth. In one case, in which the baby's heartbeat was dipping, it returned to normal as soon as the mother was upright, and she gave birth without further intervention. In this case the midwife said that squatting saved the baby from a forceps delivery.

If you want to give birth squatting following anesthesia, it is best that you have a low-dose epidural (which can always be "topped up" if necessary) so that it wears off at the end of the first stage. When you are fully dilated, your attendants will need to get you off the bed and onto the floor to support you in a standing squat. This will make it easier to bear down and greatly increase your chances of a spontaneous vaginal birth.

Using a water pool for strong labor is one of the best ways to avoid needing an epidural (see chapter 8).

FORCEPS OR VACUUM EXTRACTION

These are instruments that can be used in an emergency to help your baby out. Forceps are metal blades shaped like salad tongs. The obstetrician inserts them in the vagina on either side of the baby's head, gently assists the rotation of the head, and then applies traction to assist the delivery. A vacuum extractor attaches by suction to the baby's scalp to help ease the baby from your body. Forceps or vacuum extraction is often needed following the administration of pain-relieving techniques, such as epidural anesthesia, that weaken the power of the uterus. Occasionally an unusual presentation, a sudden rise in blood pressure, or fetal distress necessitates the use of forceps or vacuum extraction. It is difficult to assess which of these two methods is less disturbing for the baby. Vacuum extraction may be better for the mother, as it does not usually require pain medication or episiotomy, whereas forceps usually do.

If you have an active birth you are less likely to need drugs. In addition, standing, squatting, or kneeling positions greatly reduce the need for forceps or vacuum extraction. Often, after an active birth, the midwife has commented that if the woman had been lying down she may well have needed the help of forceps.

Although neither is generally used, squatting or the all-fours position is far better for these procedures than the usual reclining position. Upright postures offer these advantages:

- No compression of the blood vessels, and so more oxygen for the baby.
- Greater opening of the pelvic outlet.
- More help from gravity.
- Maximum relaxation of the perineum.
- More efficient contractions.
- Greater comfort for the mother.
- Easier access for the doctor.

ACTIVE BIRTH AND MEDICATION

Any drug you take in labor or pregnancy will travel through the placenta and enter your baby's bloodstream. All these drugs have side effects. Opponents of unmedicated childbirth say that they are not prepared to allow nature to take its course unimpeded until nature is proved to be safer than high technology. Yet almost none of the drugs used in obstetrics have been subjected to properly controlled, scientific evaluation and found to be safe in their effects on the child, at birth and in the long term. Undoubtedly there are situations where medication helps to make giving birth safer and more enjoyable. But the research that has been done clearly indicates that many drugs can have damaging effects on the mother and child and on the bonding between them after birth. Drugs should therefore be used as a backup treatment, not as routine management of normal childbirth.

When birth is active—

- There is less need for drugs.
- Discomfort and pain are less.
- The uterus functions better, so artificial stimulants are not usually necessary.
- Labors are shorter.
- The supply of oxygen to the baby is improved.
- There is less need for forceps or vacuum extraction.
- The secretion of hormones that regulate the whole process is not disrupted.

Despite the readily available studies on these findings, the majority of women in labor in this country are still confined to bed, administered drugs, and hooked up to a fetal monitor. Birth is still artificially induced and stimulated whenever pregnancy is slightly longer or labor a little slower than average. This "active management" of labor is usually done with the best of intentions to mother and child, in the name of safety. However, the routine use of medications, continuous electronic monitoring, and other features of the "high-tech" approach to labor management simply increase the number of interventive births. Given that the majority of labors are uncomplicated, there is certainly not enough evidence in favor of the drugs to justify a policy of using them routinely.

Confining a woman to bed in labor increases her need for pain-relieving drugs and artificial stimulants. Almost every woman I have worked with in active birth has reported afterwards that when she lay on her back she was astonished how much more painful the contractions were.

There are very few women who could go through labor on their backs without pain relief. Preventing a woman in labor from using her own instincts to find comfortable positions causes the need for drugs. The use of natural upright positions and immersion in water during labor makes medications seldom necessary.

"The only times the pain was extreme were those when I lay on my back for a pelvic examination. I don't think I could have managed without any drugs if I had been lying down. As when I had to in the early stages it was unbearable."

Disadvantages of Medications

It is important to be able to make an informed choice when contemplating the use of drugs. The application of drugs is very well described in the literature on childbirth, but often some of the well-known disadvantages are not mentioned.[3] Here are some examples of common drugs and their side effects:

Tranquilizers

Common among these drugs are Vistaril and Atarax. Tranquilizers can cause dizziness, confusion, and changes in blood pressure and heart rate. They pass rapidly to the baby, and may cause changes in the fetal heart-rate patterns. After birth, the baby with one of these drugs in the blood may suffer breathing or suckling problems, jaundice, diminished muscle tone, or inattentiveness.

Narcotics

These drugs, the most common of which is Demerol, reduce pain and cause drowsiness, which can sometimes help dilation if pain and tension have been slowing it (a half dose of narcotic may be effective). But—

- Narcotics depress the breathing response of the baby. A baby that has had a lot of narcotic medication may have difficulty establishing breathing and could suffer oxygen deficiency (particularly if the umbilical cord is cut immediately after birth). An antidepressant may be given to the baby to counteract the effects of the narcotic. The baby may need to be resuscitated (given oxygen and helped to breathe).
- They can disturb the baby's sucking reflex, causing problems in establishing breastfeeding that can last for several weeks or result in failure.

HOMEOPATHIC REMEDIES IN LABOR

For any complaint, there may be several homeopathic remedies from which to choose. Homeopathic physicians base their choice of remedy on individual characteristics, ascertained through detailed questioning. With many complaints, however, a certain remedy will work for most people. Low-potency homeopathic remedies are readily available from health-food stores and by mail-order (see "Resources"), and many women find them very useful. They are harmless if mischosen, and will be compatible with any other medications you may choose. You may want to have these remedies on hand for labor:

- *Arnica 30x.* For pain.
- *Aconite 30x.* For anxiety or fear.
- *Kali Phos 30x.* For exhaustion.
- *Caullophyllum 30x.* For weak, ineffectual contractions (do not take this in pregnancy).
- *Bach Rescue Remedy.* You can use this composition of flower essences throughout labor by putting a dropperful in your glass of drinking water. To help calm yourself in transition, take 10 drops in a little water, or a dropperful full strength.

Since your body can use up homeopathic remedies very rapidly in labor, you can take one dose every 30 minutes. If you wish to take more than one remedy, leave 10 minutes between.

- They are not very effective pain relievers unless they are given in large doses, in which case they often make the mother drowsy and less able to cope (particularly if they are mixed with a nausea suppressant, as is usually the case).
- If given too late in labor (after 7 centimeters dilation), narcotics can make the mother unable to focus herself properly for pushing, and they will affect the baby more by remaining in the system for several days after the birth, when the baby will not have the help of the mother's body to clear away toxins.
- They can interfere with the first contact between mother and baby by making them both drowsy.

The Caine Drugs

These drugs have names that end in *caine*—for example, Lidocaine and Marcaine.

- Used for epidurals and the other, less common regional "blocks" (spinal block and saddle block), these drugs give pain relief from the waist down in most cases, without loss of consciousness. This is especially helpful with cesareans, for which the drugs need not be administered for a prolonged period, and so have less effect on the baby than when they are used for pain relief during labor. In the case of cesareans, they facilitate the bonding of mother and child, as the mother is conscious during and immediately after the birth.
- Regional blocks reduce the muscle tone of the uterus and bladder so that they function less efficiently. A catheter is usually inserted into the urethra to help empty the bladder. The reduced efficiency of the uterus increases the need for Pitocin, forceps, or vacuum extraction (although using upright postures for the second stage, after tailing off the anesthesia at the end of the first stage, reduces the likelihood of an assisted birth).
- The mother misses the pleasurable feelings as well as the pain of childbirth, and she may regret not being able to push her baby out spontaneously.
- Regional blocks don't always work properly; sometimes they "take" on only one side. Also, the anesthesiologist may have difficulty inserting the drug, and may take a long time while the mother must remain motionless in the midst of strong contractions.
- Aftereffects such as headaches can last for a week after the birth.
- A wrongly administered regional block can result in paralysis, although this happens very rarely.
- Anesthetics lower blood pressure, which can result in less oxygen to the baby. Long periods in the reclining position, necessary for a regional block, also diminish the oxygen supply. The mother is given oxygen to help increase the supply to her baby. If the mother's blood pressure falls too low, she may become faint and dizzy.
- Although the condition of the baby after an epidural is much better than with narcotics, epidural anesthesia can cause either a nervous, jittery baby or a floppy baby who is less responsive than normal until the drugs are cleared from his or her system.

- The anesthetic enters the baby's bloodstream and brain cells within minutes, and research indicates that it could interfere with the development of the baby's brain and nervous system (see chapter 1).

When there is a complication or life is at stake, obstetric intervention and medication provide a safety net. Often medications can be combined with active birth to the advantage of mother and baby. Used routinely, however, obstetric medications can have harmful effects, both physically and psychologically.

STILLBIRTH

In the case of a stillbirth, active birth has many advantages. Giving birth spontaneously, without the use of drugs, may help the mother to feel that she has gained something from the experience and that she may be able to use her knowledge again in a future birth. Also, if she delivers in the kneeling position, her attendants have time to prepare her to see and hold the baby. She will recover faster and feel physically well, which will help her to cope with the emotional pain that is inevitable after such an experience. Additionally, if the father of the baby is with her, they may both benefit from sharing the birth and the grieving.

> *"Looking back over my two pregnancies, my overwhelming impression is one of peaceful well-being. In both cases I started exercising regularly at about three months and experienced a growing satisfaction as I reached towards my body's potential. My first pregnancy sadly ended in a stillbirth, but, on being encouraged to use all the positive elements gained from the classes, I tried for and achieved as good and natural a birth as possible. I feel sure that this helped enormously towards my ability to accept and live with the pain of the loss. How glad I was on giving birth to my second baby that I had had this first good experience."*

A NOTE TO THE BIRTH ATTENDANT

If you are presented with this book by a woman who would like to put its teaching into practice, I hope you will enjoy helping her to do so. The practice of active birth should help to make the atmosphere within the hospital more homelike for those families who prefer, or for medical reasons choose, to have their babies in the hospital. It is possible to combine some of the psychological advantages of home with the security of the hospital by making a few basic changes. What is mainly needed is the right attitude towards the woman.

"My doctor's innate confidence in the normal workings of a healthy body was a real factor for calm and confidence both during my pregnancy and at the birth."

"Both the midwife and her student were friendly and said, 'Do whatever you like.' Ditto the nun in charge of the labor ward, whom I knew from the time of Michael's birth, since she had been on the maternity ward. She remembered and welcomed us, and offered to put a blanket on the floor if I wanted to go on using my cushion."

It is essential that the mother in labor should not be considered as a patient. The attendants should regard themselves as her guests, there to assist her in giving birth, which to her is a very special occasion in her sexual, social, and emotional life. While carefully observing the progress of mother and baby, the attendants should try not to disturb the natural process of the birth. Interference should be kept to the minimum necessary to ensure safety. This means that both mother and attendant will rely more upon their instincts and intuition. Research has shown that, whether at home or in the hospital, when birth is regarded as natural and instinctive and interference is minimal, safety statistics are impressively better (for example, in Holland and Pithiviers, France). With active birth, the art of midwifery comes back into its own, and attendants can become more spontaneous and flexible in their approach.

The Birth Room

Here are some helpful things to have in the room in which women labor and give birth:

- Curtains that can be drawn to darken the room,
- Dimmers on the lights,
- A beanbag chair or pile of large cushions with attractive, colorful covers,
- A comfortable stool for support in the squatting position—perhaps a wooden birthstool,
- A comfortable armchair,
- A cassette tape recorder (or suggest that women bring their own),
- A hand-held heart monitor (stethoscope or Doptone),
- A hot-water bottle,
- A crockpot, and
- A washable nonslip yoga mat for the mother to stand or squat on for the delivery.

Water is so helpful to mothers in labor that the hospital birth room should include a bathroom and shower, or at least free access to those nearby. A small pool, or a double-size bath (rather deeper than usual), is extremely helpful.

If there is a bed in the birth room, it should not be too high or narrow. A low platform with a firm mattress is most comfortable. Remember that the furniture in a room suggests how one should behave in it. If the first thing a woman sees on entering the room is a delivery bed, she immediately feels she ought to get onto it, and is already a "patient," robbed of her power.

Assisting the Mother

Midwifery is, to a large extent, a social profession—you are working with a growing family or with a couple who are becoming a family. To the woman in labor, the attendant is extremely important. If the mother feels the attendant to be a friend, someone she can totally trust and relax with, the labor will progress better, and the birth will be a

A NOTE TO THE BIRTH ATTENDANT (cont.)

better experience for all concerned. Naturally, the primary concern to the birth attendant is the safe delivery of a healthy baby to a healthy mother. But by encouraging mothers to follow their own instincts—by showing that *you* trust *them*—you will help them to give birth in a way that is satisfying as well as safe. Your belief in the natural birth process will make them feel confident—especially when the going gets tough.

If you work in a busy hospital where birth is a daily occurrence, you need to remind yourself that, for the family concerned, birth happens only once or a few times in a lifetime. The woman needs to feel that she is the center of what is happening, that this is her day. Her privacy, and the profound and intimate nature of what she is experiencing, should be respected at all times.

> *"I was taken straight into the labor ward and was given a big cushion so as to save my own from being soiled. Only one midwife was present, and she let me do what I wanted, helping me squat, advising me on breathing, and massaging me."*

It will help the mother greatly to feel at home if she is encouraged to use her body freely during labor and delivery, and to give birth on the floor if she chooses to. A clean sheet, a firm mattress, or a nonslip yoga mat can be placed on the floor. The usual sterile paper pad or an absorbent towel can be placed between her legs when the birth is imminent.

In strong labor and transition, the mother needs privacy in order to surrender and open up. Distractions should be minimized, especially as the second stage is starting. Routine examination to check dilation is usually unnecessary (see page 179). In the second stage women rarely need to be given instructions but should be encouraged to let go, pushing when they feel like it. It is not necessary to use the delivery position until the head is actually crowning (see page 139).

In labor, necessary checks on the dilation and fetal heart can be done, with the minimum of disruption to the mother, in a position in which she is comfortable. It is important to bear in mind that a dilating cervix is the most tender and vulnerable part of a woman's body.

It is of great comfort to some women, and their husbands, if they can bring a close female friend or relative to the birth if they choose to do so. The emotional support is doubled, and this also helps the staff.

If the woman has other children, it is advisable to allow them in very soon after the birth (within the first hour) to meet the new baby and reunite with their mother. Immediately after the birth, you can help the new relationship get off to a good start by doing the essential checking of the infant while he or she is in the mother's arms. Then the family should be left alone together, with the midwife discreetly nearby, for at least half an hour, and the mother should be brought something to drink. The baby should be left undressed but warmly wrapped in a soft flannel sheet to facilitate skin-to-skin contact. More detailed examination of the baby and stitching of tears can be done after this half hour, if all is well.

Separation after a momentous occasion like a birth can be traumatic for a couple. Allowing the father to stay with the mother for the first night or the first few days offers great psychological advantages.

> *"When everyone had gone and I lay bathed and clean between clean sheets, with my husband asleep on one side of me and my little baby in my arms, I felt a supreme sense of peace and rightness with the world and the laws of nature."*

The exercises recommended for mothers in this book can also help attendants, who need to be comfortable in kneeling and crouching positions if they are to assist a woman who is squatting. It is helpful to wear trousers for an active birth. Some midwives find "scrub suits" ideal for this purpose. Take care to protect your back while bending or squatting; bend your knees or use a very low stool. The physical therapist at your hospital may be able to help you find suitable stress-free positions.

8 | Water Birth

SO FAR WE HAVE CONSIDERED THE EFFECT OF GRAVITY
on the normal physiology of the birth process. We have observed the
disadvantages of defying gravity by lying flat or remaining immobile in
the semireclining position, and we have considered how you can position
your body in harmony with both gravity and your own instincts. When
you enter a pool of warm water in labor, the buoyancy of the water reduces
the effect of gravity, allowing you to float freely or change positions, more
or less weightless. Many women feel attracted to water in labor, and find
that immersion in a warm pool is a helpful way to relax and surrender to
the involuntary forces at work in their bodies, and to ease the pain and
discomfort of strong contractions. Some women choose to remain in a
pool during the second stage, and to give birth in the water. The value of
using warm water during labor and birth is increasingly being recognized.
Immersion in water will, I hope, become a more popular option in the
coming decades, so that many more women will have a pool available
for their use in the birthing environment.

THE HISTORY OF WATER BIRTH

Water is our original element. In the first nine months in the womb the fetus develops in the aquatic environment of the amniotic fluid. Like a miniature sea, the waters of the womb provide the ideal medium for the growing baby, protecting him or her from shock or injury. Bathing in water continues to play an important role throughout the child's and adult's life as a way to relax and relieve tension. Water is used therapeutically, in hydrotherapy, and also for purification or sanctification in religious rituals all over the world.

In the past few decades there has been increasing interest in the use of water during pregnancy, birth, and infancy. Along with yoga, swimming is an ideal way to exercise in pregnancy. Free from the full force of gravity, the mother can enjoy a pleasant and relieving feeling of lightness, as well as greater ease of movement, while enhancing her cardiovascular fitness. Midwives have known for years that a warm bath can relax a mother and speed the progress of her labor.

The idea of a laboring woman entering a pool of water deep enough for her to be fully immersed, and the possibility of actually giving birth under water, was first explored fully by the Soviet researcher Igor Tjarkovsky in the 1960s (although his work was preceded by that of several other Russian researchers).[1] Later in the same decade, the French obstetrician Frederick Leboyer introduced the idea of bathing newborn babies in warm water immediately after they had been born, to help them to acclimatize gradually to life outside their mother's womb.

Another pioneer of water birth is Michel Odent, who first thought of using warm water as a way to ease pain during labor. He installed a simple inflatable pool adjoining the "primitive" birthing room at the general hospital in Pithiviers, France, in 1977, and by 1983 thousands of women had used the pool during labor, and about a hundred of them had given birth under water.[2]

Odent emphasizes that in his view the goal is not necessarily to give birth under water; rather, the warm water is a tool to facilitate labor. In his experience, most women prefer to get out for the second stage. (At the Garden Hospital, a surprising 30 to 50 percent of women who use a pool in labor stay in the water to give birth. The number of water births increases, I've found, as midwives gain confidence. But I agree with Odent that giving birth in water should not be the goal.) The main use of

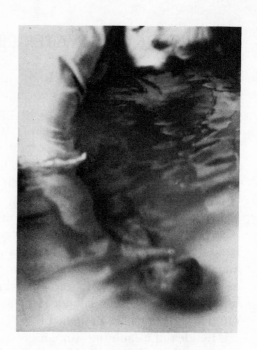

Michel Odent lifts a baby born in
water in the birth pool at Pithiviers.

the pool is to reduce pain and enhance relaxation so the mother can get through labor without any medications.

Odent discovered that the pool was especially useful for women who were having long and painful labors (particularly with backache) and who were having difficulty progressing beyond 5 centimeters dilation. After the woman entered the pool, the midwife would dim the lights, and usually the warm water would help the mother to reach full dilation within a couple of hours.

When the mother gave birth in the water, Odent observed, being in the pool seemed to enhance the first contact between mother and baby. The mother seemed to express her emotions more easily, and the baby relaxed more and was easier to hold. Odent could identify no special risks in either labor or birth in water.[3] "It should be possible," Odent says, "for any conventional hospital to have a pool situated close to the birthing room and operating theatre. . . . Immersion in warm water is an efficient, easy, and economical way to reduce the use of drugs and the rate of intervention in parturition."[4]

Since the early 1980s, the use of water pools has spread, and many groups of people have reported similarly positive results, notably in the

United Kingdom, North America, Belgium, Scandinavia, Australia, and New Zealand.[5] In the United Kingdom, 30 state hospitals had installed water pools by January 1992, and more than 100 portable pools were in constant use. Many U.S. hospitals, too, are installing pools in birthing rooms.

Giving birth in water appeals to many parents as a way to ease the trauma of birth for their babies and to ensure a gentle transition from the protected watery world of the womb to the full force of gravity on land. Studies of water pool use are still being undertaken, but so far the evidence strongly confirms that a water pool is a powerful and harmless aid to women giving birth actively—an aid that helps to reduce even further the need for drugs and interventions. Women who have used water pools are very enthusiastic indeed about the relief they have enjoyed in the water. Birth attendants, too, are impressed with the results of using water pools, which they find make their work easier and more enjoyable.

CONSIDERING A WATER BIRTH

When considering the possibility of using water for your baby's birth, avoid having too many preconceptions or rigid expectations. It is impossible to know ahead of time what will happen. You may find that you do not feel attracted to water at all, or that an unexpected complication makes the use of a pool inappropriate. Perhaps the birth will happen so fast that you won't need the pool. Or you may intend to use the pool for your labor only and find that you end up giving birth in the water. Some mothers who planned to use pools for birth, and then didn't in the end, have derived great pleasure from the pools in the days following birth.

Whatever happens, birth is an adventure, and it is reassuring to have a water pool available to use as and when appropriate.

PRACTICALITIES

The water pool to be used for labor and birth should be large enough and deep enough to allow for a variety of positions and the possibility of another person entering the water. It is best when the water is deep enough so that the mother is immersed up to just above her breasts when sitting. A variety of water pools are now available for rent or purchase, and some of these, designed to be portable, can be set up temporarily in your own home or in a hospital (see "Resources"). It is important that the pool be equipped with an efficient pump, a heater, and a thermostat. A water thermometer and a large plastic strainer to clear the water are important extras. The edge of the pool needs to be padded so there is a soft wall to lean against, and a variety of water cushions is useful.

The water temperature should be approximately 99°F, about body temperature and comfortably warm. If the water is too warm or too cool, this may affect labor. Ordinary tap water is quite suitable, and no additives are necessary, although some people add salt to the water to reach a degree of salinity about that of amniotic fluid (1 generous tablespoon salt per gallon of water). The pool needs to be cleaned beforehand with a mild disinfectant, unless disposable liners are provided to contain the water.

PREPARING FOR A WATER BIRTH

The yoga-based exercises described in this book are ideal preparation for birth in or out of water. Additionally, it is very beneficial to swim during pregnancy and to spend time relaxing in water everyday, especially in the last three months. Specific water exercises are not essential, but you will find that several of the postures in this book can be practiced under water as well. Gentle breaststroke and backstroke are very pleasurable, and floating on your back is blissfully relaxing, as the buoyancy gives relief from the weight of pregnancy.

Many pregnant women enjoy luxuriating in the bathtub—sometimes more than once a day. The addition of four or five drops of essential oil, such as lavender, tangerine, rose, or jasmine, can be very relaxing.

USING WATER FOR LABOR

It is generally thought that the best time to enter the pool is midway through labor, at about 5 centimeters dilation, when the contractions are becoming very intense. (It has been observed that entering the pool earlier can sometimes slow contractions and prolong labor.) While this is a useful guideline, it should not be used as a fast rule. If you feel an irresistible urge to enter the water, this should not be denied.

Check the water temperature before entering the pool; make sure it is not too warm. It is helpful to have the room darkened and to maintain a calm and peaceful atmosphere with attendants reduced to only those who are essential. The nurse or midwife should listen to the fetal heart just before you enter the pool; this can be repeated from time to time, if necessary, with a small, hand-held ultrasound heart monitor or a traditional obstetric stethoscope. Monitoring can easily be done while you sit, stand, or kneel in the pool, or you can float to the surface with someone gently supporting your lower back.

In the warm water you can relax and let go, breathing calmly and deeply through the contractions, moving and changing positions to make yourself comfortable. It is possible to kneel against the edge, to squat, to semisit, or to float as you please, and from time to time you may enjoy immersing your whole body, including your head. You will find that the water allows you to take sensual pleasure in your body, to forget what is happening around you, and to surrender to your instinctive urges. Most women find that their perception of pain changes in the water; it becomes much easier to accept the intensity of the contractions.

Once you have had a chance to relax in the water, labor will probably progress quite rapidly. It occasionally happens, however, that contractions slow down and become less intense. If this situation persists, it is best to leave the pool and make use of gravity. After you move around for a while outside the pool, using upright resting positions, rhythmic contractions should soon build up again, and labor will probably reestablish itself.

Should your membranes rupture there is no need to leave or change the water, as the amniotic fluid and blood from a "show" are sterile. Michel Odent reported, "We had no infectious complications, even where the membranes were already broken."[6] There is no evidence of an increased infection rate in any other birth center where water births take place; in fact, the use of a water pool may reduce the risk of infection, especially in a hospital, where infection from foreign bacteria in the air is more likely.

A water pool has other advantages in the hospital environment. It may increase a woman's sense of privacy, giving her a space of her own to relax and feel safe in, where she can be less aware of what is going on around her. Immersion in warm water tends to lower blood pressure raised by anxiety, and it certainly reduces pain.[7] This is due partially to the loss of the effects of gravity and partially, perhaps, to a fall in the production of catecholamines (stress hormones like adrenaline) and a rise in the secretion of endorphins (hormones that are natural relaxants and pain relievers).

Many hospitals, midwives, and doctors who are apprehensive about actual birth taking place under water are open to the use of a water pool for labor. The provision of a pool for the latter part of the first stage is a completely safe and harmless way to facilitate labor, and it provides a risk-free alternative to painkilling medications or epidurals.

If a pool is not available, any access to water is helpful. It is possible, for example, to kneel in an ordinary bathtub with your partner sponging warm water soothingly over your back. Try to make the water as deep as possible and comfortably warm. Alternatively, standing or squatting in the shower with the warm water running down your back, or even sponging and splashing yourself with water from the hand basin, can help you. Sometimes just the sound of a tap running can stimulate contractions and help a woman let go of inhibitions. Warm and cold compresses, spray bottles and hot-water bottles, ice, and natural sponges rinsed out in cold water are all tried and tested labor aids.

GIVING BIRTH UNDER WATER

Your labor may progress so quickly that there is no time to leave the pool and your baby is simply born into the water. Perhaps you will deliberately choose to stay in the water for the birth, or you may well feel like getting out. It is wise not to decide ahead of time whether your baby will be born in the water or not. Sometimes it is sensible or necessary to leave the pool, and take advantage of the help of gravity or a cooler atmosphere, to facilitate the second stage. A doctor or midwife to whom water birth is new may be reluctant to deliver a baby in water, although confidence usually comes with experience.

Reasons for leaving the pool might be—

- You feel that you want to leave the water.
- The second stage is prolonged.
- There are signs of possible fetal distress—for example, meconium (the baby's fecal matter) is released into the water.
- The baby is a breech. (Some maintain that the warmth of the water might reduce the risk of a breech baby "breathing," and hence the placenta separating, before the head emerges. But few breech babies

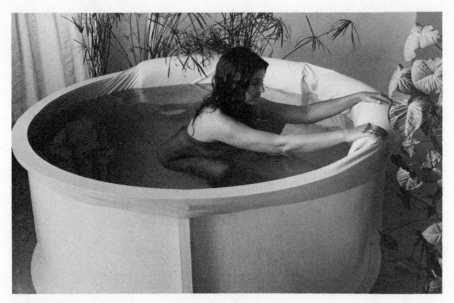

Kneeling or squatting in the birth pool during strong labor helps to relieve pain and enhances contractions.

have been born under water. Given the increased risk of a breech birth, it is generally considered wiser to make optimal use of gravity in the standing squat position.)

- The baby is unusually large and not descending well in the second stage. In this case the use of gravity outside the pool will be more effective in helping the birth.
- You have twins. Since there is more risk with a twin birth—especially for the second twin—it is considered safer for the mother to give birth out of water.
- The placenta may not be functioning at its best, although there is no sign of fetal distress. In this case water may possibly be used to facilitate the labor, but birth in the supported standing squat is preferable.

It is common for the mother to excrete some fecal matter as the baby's head descends and compresses the bowel, and as the anal sphincter muscle relaxes prior to birth. Some mothers choose to have an enema in early labor to prevent this occurring, but it might happen anyway. If it occurs in the water, the debris should simply be removed immediately with an ordinary plastic strainer. The excretion of fecal matter is a common occurrence in births both in and out of water, and there is no evidence to show that it contaminates the water sufficiently to contribute any risk of infection. On the contrary, in the United Kingdom there have been no reports of infectious complications with water births.

Positions for Underwater Birth

You can give birth in the water in a variety of positions, changing from one to another spontaneously. You can kneel in an all-fours position over the edge of the pool, with the baby emerging from behind. Alternatively, you can squat in the water, holding onto the sides for support. You can squat unsupported; this is much easier in the water than on the floor or bed. Your partner can enter the pool to support you, or he or she can sit outside the pool on a low stool or a beanbag chair and support you from behind.[8] You might choose a semisitting position.

Your midwife or doctor will probably not enter the pool. Attendants in the United Kingdom, often wearing the cotton trousers and top worn in operating rooms, enter the pool only if necessary. It is usually quite easy to observe what is happening from the side, and the danger to the attendant of cross-infection from the AIDS or hepatitis virus may be a concern. (Although there is yet no evidence of these diseases being transmitted through water, a few hospitals have been asking women who wish to use a water pool to be tested in pregnancy.)

The Second Stage

Your baby's head may crown very quickly, or it may be some time before the baby is ready to be born. Eventually the head will appear and begin to show through your vagina. You may find that in water it is easier to release your feelings without inhibition; most mothers cry out freely at this stage. If you feel like it, you can use your own hands to sense what is happening and help the baby to emerge. Because the warmth of the water helps to soften the perineal tissues, it is very unusual for a bad tear to occur during a water birth (midwives have observed that there is less damage to the perineum even when the mother has only labored in water). There is usually no need for the attendant to do anything at all as the baby emerges gently into the water. If the body of the baby is not expelled in the contraction following the emergence of the head, the midwife or doctor can gently assist.

The water in the pool will almost certainly become quite bloody soon after the birth. There is no danger of infection, as this blood, from the lining of the womb, is sterile.

The Third Stage

Once the baby is born, the midwife or doctor will check to see if the cord is around the baby's neck, and simply unravel it if it is. If the cord is long enough, the baby may well float up to the surface, or you, your partner, or the attendant may gently lift the baby up. There is no hurry to lift the baby out of the water, but this should be done within the first minute or so after the birth. It is dangerous to keep the baby immersed longer than this, since the baby's first need is to start breathing independently after birth. In the brief time the baby is under water, the placental circulation continues and the baby receives blood and oxygen through the umbilical

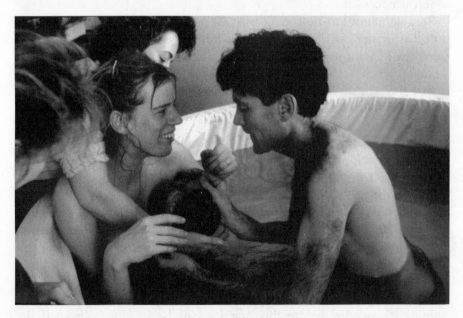

Immediately after birth under water, the father gently lifts the baby to the surface and passes him to his mother.

cord. The placental circulation will cease only after the baby's breathing is established.

Dolphins, porpoises, and whales—mammals who give birth in water—usually push their young to the surface to breathe within the first few minutes. The baby's breathing is stimulated by the cooler temperature of the atmosphere on its skin; breathing will not occur until the baby emerges into the cool air. Because human babies react the same way, it is important that the room not be overheated.

Once he or she is gently lifted up, you can cuddle the baby in your arms, close to your breast, with the face out of the water while the body may remain submerged. Water-born babies rarely have any difficulty establishing breathing; the cooler temperature on the baby's face is enough to trigger the breathing reflex. Very occasionally a baby needs suctioning to clear the nasal passages; this can be done while the baby's body is still in the water. It is not wise to cut the cord yet, as the baby is still benefiting from two sources of oxygen. In the rare circumstance that the baby doesn't breathe, it is wise to take the baby gently out of the pool into a cooler atmosphere. This will trigger the breathing reflex, and oxygen can be given if necessary.

It is wonderful to hold your baby in your arms in the water and look into his or her eyes for the very first time. It is best to be in a vertical position, kneeling or sitting upright, so you can hold the baby comfortably at breast level. You will probably find that your baby has a strong rooting reflex and will soon be turning its head to search for the breast. It is best to turn the baby towards you "belly to belly" to assist the first sucking. It is quite safe to remain in the water until your uterus begins to contract again to expel the placenta (usually 10 to 20 minutes).

Close attention should be paid to the cord. A decrease in pulse, as well as strong uterine contractions when the baby sucks, indicates the placenta is ready to separate. Then it is time to stand up slowly and leave the pool. It is generally considered safer to stand up or to leave the pool before the placenta is expelled than after, to prevent the possibility of water embolism (water entering the bloodstream through any blood vessels that are still open inside the womb). This is a sensible precaution, although no incidence of water embolism in a water birth has ever been recorded. (The Garden Hospital allows delivery of the placenta in the water, but further studies are needed before this practice can be recommended.) If the placenta unexpectedly separates before you leave the pool, simply stand up slowly as soon as you realize what has happened. The cord can be cut just before you leave the pool, although you need not cut it until after delivery of the placenta.

Your attendants can help you to leave the pool and have warm towels ready for you and the baby. A warm terrycloth robe is useful to put on when you get out. This is the time to increase the temperature in the room; an efficient portable heater should be available so that the room can be made very warm at this point. Once you are outside the pool you can stand up or squat to deliver the placenta, and then sit down upright for a while. Make sure that both you and baby are warm and comfortable while you continue to welcome your baby and enjoy the first breast-feeding.

You can give the baby a warm bath after the birth if you wish to continue water immersion or if the baby seems cold, but the warmth of your body is quite sufficient. Once the midwife has checked your perineum and has had a good look at the baby, you will probably feel like relaxing comfortably in bed with your baby tucked in warmly beside you, close to the familiar warmth of your body.

AFTER THE BIRTH

If the pool is available to you in the days following the birth, you may enjoy spending time in the pool, and this pleasure can be shared with other family members. Siblings take great pleasure in holding their newborn sister or brother in the warm water, and the baby will enjoy the freedom of being in the familiar watery medium while getting to know you and the rest of the family, and exploring the world all around. Ensure that the room temperature is very warm, and keep the lighting subdued for the first day or two. The water in the pool should of course be changed, and the pool should be comfortably warm, but not hot. Newborn babies dislike sudden exposure to the elements, so take care to undress the baby slowly, in a very warm room, and to hold the baby against your body, covered by a warm towel. Enter the pool slowly so the baby makes a gradual transition into the water; the same applies when leaving the pool. It can be blissful to breastfeed your baby while in the pool, making sure the baby's body is submerged to the shoulders. The baby can remain in the water for up to 30 to 45 minutes to begin with, if this feels comfortable, and gradually the time can be extended.

TIPS FOR THE ATTENDANT

Few midwives and doctors have yet been trained to use water during labor and birth. Here are answers to some common queries.

- Although British midwives have discovered that their hand-held ultrasound monitors can be used under water without getting ruined, special waterproof ones are now available from most suppliers.
- If there is any difficulty in getting a monitor reading under water, the mother can easily float up to the surface, where a hand placed under her lower back will support her comfortably. If her partner is in the pool he or she can assist by sitting behind the mother and supporting her lower back. Alternatively, she can stand up or sit on the edge of the pool.
- Essential internal examinations can be done quite easily underwater, with the mother on all fours. The descent of the head can be checked in any position by feeling.
- The delivery usually needs no assistance, but the midwife or doctor should be ready if necessary.
- The midwife or doctor rarely needs to enter the pool for a water birth. Further research is needed to ensure the doctor or midwife's safety from cross-infection with the AIDS or hepatitis virus, but in the meantime attendants should be sure they have no open wounds on their hands or arms, and use rubber gloves as a precaution.
- Unless the second stage progresses well, the mother should leave the pool for the birth.
- After a birth in the water, hold the baby belly down while passing it to the mother, to help the fluids to drain.
- When the cord pulsation ceases, it is time for the mother and baby to leave the pool.
- It is important to learn how to bend to avoid backache. A stool is helpful.

Contact the Active Birth Centre (see "Resources") for details of training or further information.

9 | After the Birth

YOUR BODY AFTER BIRTH

After the birth, you may be surprised to find that each time your baby sucks at the breast your uterus contracts. These contractions, known as "afterpains," may be painful at first, like strong menstrual cramps, especially if this is your second or subsequent child. They are helping your uterus to retract back into the pelvis and return to its normal shape and size. After a few days the pains will gradually stop and will be replaced by a feeling of pleasure and well-being as you breastfeed your baby.

You may be fortunate after the birth to find that your perineum is intact with no tear. In this case there may be very little soreness or tenderness, and recovery will be quick. Or you may have a graze, which requires no stitching, or a tear or episiotomy that needs to be repaired. Stitching is usually done soon after you have welcomed your baby, and a local anesthetic is used so that you feel no pain. Generally, a natural tear will heal rapidly in a day or so and cause little scarring. It is advisable to use the healing and antiseptic herbal bath (see page 218) for a day or two after the birth to ensure a good recovery and prevent infection.

HERBAL BATH FOR AFTER BIRTH

For a soothing, healing antiseptic miracle for perineal tears, grazes, or episiotomies, take three heads of garlic. Do not peel them, but prick them all over with a fork. Put them in a large saucepan with a generous handful each of shepherd's purse, uva-ursi, and comfrey (all available from good herb and health-food stores). Fill the pan with water, and bring to a boil. Simmer gently for ½ to ¾ hour.

Remove the garlic from the pan, and let it cool enough to handle. With a fork, squeeze the juice from the garlic into the pan, and let the liquid cool. Strain the liquid into a large jar. Pour half the liquid into a shallow warm bath, and sit in the bath for a while.

Do this once or twice daily.

If you find there is stinging when you urinate, pour a large jugful of warm water between your legs at the same time, or use a squirt bottle. Pat dry afterwards with a clean towel. You might dab the scar with homeopathic calendula tincture, which is antiseptic and promotes healing (use it undiluted, or dilute 10 drops in 2 tablespoons previously boiled water). Allow yourself to dry before dressing. Do not use ointment or cream, as the moistness could dissolve the stitches too rapidly. Use a child's swimming ring to sit on if you are uncomfortable. Later, when the wound is healing (at the itching stage), apply a little vitamin E oil after bathing to prevent scarring and promote healing.

Bleeding from the uterus (known as *lochia*) will continue for some time—like a long period—gradually lessening, until all the blood-rich lining of the uterus has been shed. Use sanitary napkins rather than tampons, as the latter may cause infection.

In the hours after giving birth, you will probably find it impossible to fall asleep. You need to bask in the afterglow of the birth, and to go over all that has happened, before weariness takes over and you fall asleep. Your baby, too, will probably be very alert for a few hours, and then fall into a profound sleep.

It is best to keep your baby in close body contact with you for several days and to enjoy an extended "babymoon," with few visitors for the first week after birth. At least a few quiet days getting to know one another as a family will be invaluable. Your partner will need time and peace to "bond" with the baby, too, as both of you learn how to respond to his or her basic needs. For the first day or two you will probably find that the very special atmosphere that follows the birth continues, but it is very easy to shatter this atmosphere with insensitive intrusion. It is well worth making careful preparation beforehand for these first special days. Many parents who do report a postnatal euphoria that continues for a week or two and certainly helps them to acclimatize to early parenthood.

STARTING TO BREASTFEED

With the prospect of giving birth ahead, women often give little thought to breastfeeding. Sometimes, especially after an active birth, breastfeeding follows with little or no difficulty. More often than not, however, there is a lot to learn. The first week or two can be quite challenging.

It is helpful to understand some basic physiology before you start. In the first day or two after birth your breasts produce a substance known as *colostrum*. This is a thick, yellowish liquid that you may have noticed on your nipples in the last weeks of pregnancy. This wonderful fluid is the perfect first food for your baby. It is highly nutritious and contains valuable antibodies that fortify your baby's immune system for the future and help to protect your baby from bacteria in the environment. Since it also has a laxative quality, it clears your baby's digestive tract, preparing it to absorb milk in the days to come. It will help to clear the *meconium* from your baby's bowel. This is a sticky, dark green substance that collects in your baby's bowel during pregnancy. After birth, within a day or two, your baby begins to defecate, and the first meconium appears. Gradually, with the help of colostrum, all the meconium passes, and by the third or fourth day it is replaced by soft yellow stools.

An important reason to keep your baby close to you in the first few days is to encourage the baby to take in as much of the colostrum as needed. Michel Odent, in his book *Primal Health*, stresses the need for the baby to consume "huge quantities" of colostrum.[1] Because the baby's sucking stimulates colostrum production, it is important not to limit sucking time. Supplemental water or glucose (sugar) water is rarely necessary for a healthy baby fed in this way, and weight loss is usually negligible.

Proper sucking will also stimulate the release of the first milk. In the hours before milk "comes in" your baby may be a little fretful and impatient. This is especially common with big babies, who sometimes seem to be ravenous just before the milk comes in. A few drops of pure water on a clean teaspoon will help to quench the baby's thirst. The milk usually comes in within two to four days after the birth, and the day it does is often a little difficult. Your breasts will probably become engorged—that is, swollen and hot.

Engorgement can be very uncomfortable, but it usually lasts only about 24 hours. You may also find that you are very emotional on the day the milk comes in, and you may need to ensure that you have private time to rest and relax without visitors until this phase passes. It may be more difficult for your baby to latch on to the breasts while they are engorged.

To ease the discomfort of engorgement—

- Before feeding, lie on your belly in the bath and massage your breasts gently towards the nipple to express a little milk into the warm water.
- Stand under a warm shower with the water coming down onto your breasts.
- Apply cold compresses for a short while after feeding.
- Try taking the homeopathic remedy Belladonna 6x every half an hour until symptoms ease, if engorgement is very bad.
- Try using a long scarf instead of a bra. In many traditional societies midwives bind the breasts this way. Make the scarf firm and supportive but not too tight, and wrap it around the neck halter-style to secure it. A sports bra may also be comfortable.

HOW DOES BREASTFEEDING WORK?

The first principle of breastfeeding is supply and demand. The amount your baby sucks will determine the supply of milk. Your baby can increase the supply by sucking more (which is what is happening on days when sucking seems endless). Milk is produced in little cells that are arranged in clusters within the breast; they look a bit like miniature bunches of grapes. When your baby sucks, signals go via nerve endings to your pituitary gland in the brain, which releases the hormone oxytocin. The oxytocin makes the milk-producing cells contract and release the milk (it also makes your uterus contract at the same time). The milk is ejected into little ducts that carry it to the *ampullae*, the reservoirs just behind the areola. You can feel these as little lumps surrounding the base of the areola (the dark area around your nipple). From there the milk is ejected via the tiny openings in your nipples. At first there may seem to be far too much milk, but gradually the amount your baby sucks will determine the right supply.

You may feel the "let-down reflex" as a tingling sensation in the breast; however, it may take a few weeks for this sensation to develop. The milk may let down as soon as you even think of feeding, or only after your baby has sucked for a minute or two. Therefore it is vital not to take your baby off the breast after just a couple of minutes, as mothers are often wrongly advised to do. If you remove the baby before the milk lets down, production will be inhibited and the milk supply may eventually dry up.

It is best not to time feeding at all. Allow your baby to suck until he or she is satisfied; then offer the other breast. It is important to let your baby empty the breast at each feeding, as the milk changes consistency through a feeding, and the richest milk comes at the end. Babies vary greatly in the amount of time they take to complete a feeding, but usually they fall blissfully asleep at the end.

Feed your baby according to demand. At first it may seem as if you're spending all your time breastfeeding, but remember that your baby has been used to continuous feeding in the womb. Gradually a pattern of feeding and digesting will emerge.

To prevent nipple soreness, position your baby correctly at the breast:

1. Sit upright in a comfortable chair or in bed. Soon you will also be able to breastfeed lying on your side, with your baby cradled beside you (if you have had a cesarean you will need to start in this position).

2. Make sure you are holding your baby comfortably "belly to belly"—that is, with the baby's mouth facing the nipple and his or her body facing towards yours.

3. To help your baby "latch on" properly, wait for the baby to open his or her mouth wide. This may require a bit of tantalizing: touch the nipple to the baby's lower lip.

4. When the mouth is wide open, draw the baby towards the breast, using your free hand, if necessary, to help offer the breast to the baby. Make sure that your baby takes in a good part of the areola as well as the nipple. The part underneath the nipple is most important; it should be mostly taken into the baby's mouth, unless you have very large areolae.

Remember that your baby feeds from the whole breast and not from just the nipple. Your baby must "milk" the breast by massaging the ampullae—the milk reservoirs behind the areola—with rhythmic movements of the lower jaw. Once the baby has drawn the nipple and areola into his or her mouth, the massaging movement of the baby's jaw and tongue stimulates the ejection of the milk. When a baby is latched on properly, the nipple reaches right to the back of the soft palate (to get an idea of how this works try sucking your thumb for a moment).

If your baby is latching on properly, most breastfeeding problems will be prevented. Some discomfort and nipple soreness can be expected, but continued feeding should "break in" the nipples, and soreness will pass.

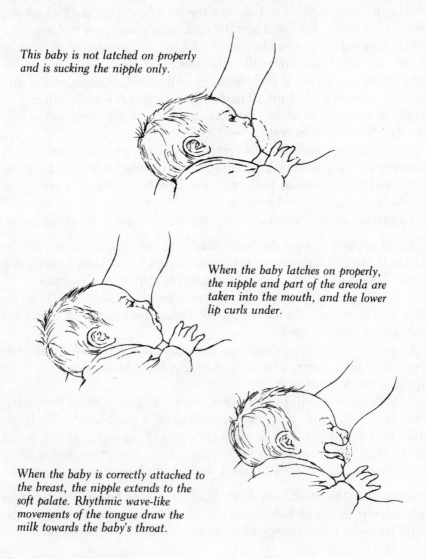

This baby is not latched on properly and is sucking the nipple only.

When the baby latches on properly, the nipple and part of the areola are taken into the mouth, and the lower lip curls under.

When the baby is correctly attached to the breast, the nipple extends to the soft palate. Rhythmic wave-like movements of the tongue draw the milk towards the baby's throat.

If difficulties arise, contact a lactation consultant or a breastfeeding counselor from La Leche League or the Nursing Mothers Counsel as soon as possible (see "Resources"). It is wise to make contact with a breastfeeding counselor near to you before the birth, especially if you are having twins.

BREAST CARE

The following advice should be helpful:

- In late pregnancy massage your breasts and nipples with almond oil after bathing. Read a good book on breastfeeding (see "Recommended Reading").
- Never use soap on your breasts, as this removes natural lubricants.
- Don't wash your breasts between feedings. Milk contains natural antiseptics and one bath or shower a day is sufficient to ensure cleanliness.
- After a feeding allow your breast to air-dry, and then massage a little pure almond oil into the nipples.

NEWBORN JAUNDICE

About half of all babies get mild jaundice in the first week of life. Their skin and the whites of their eyes turn yellowish. The yellow pigment is bilirubin, which the baby's liver is unable to completely break down during the first few days after birth. Premature babies are more prone to jaundice, and some experts believe that clamping the cord before delivery of the placenta increases the incidence of jaundice.[2]

The jaundiced baby should be put to the breast often, as he or she needs the fluid. (There is no advantage in giving water, or water and glucose, if the baby is nursing well.) Sunlight on the baby's bare skin is also helpful.

If the baby is alert and nursing well, the jaundice is probably mild and harmless. In extreme cases, however, phototherapy is needed. Portable "bili-lights" are available in some areas for phototherapy treatment at home.

- Wear a well-fitted cotton bra. Choose one that opens in front.
- Use washable or disposable breast pads that do not contain plastic, and change them frequently.
- If soreness occurs, apply homeopathic calendula cream after feedings. This will not harm your baby.
- Expose sore nipples to fresh air as much as possible. Mild sunshine for a short period will help.
- When you must remove your baby from the breast, break the suction first, by inserting your little finger into the corner of your baby's mouth.

BREASTFEEDING IN THE MONTHS TO COME

After a week or two, breastfeeding your baby should become a pleasure that nourishes both of you. Breast milk is the perfect food for your baby, providing exactly the right nutrients throughout the first year. Although you may introduce solid food when your baby is around four to six months old, breast milk should form the mainstay of your baby's diet for twelve months or longer, if possible. There is no food for your baby as complete in nutrients as breast milk. Baby formula made from cow's milk can make an adequate substitute, if necessary, for it has been formulated to resemble human breast milk as closely as possible. However, it cannot entirely imitate the dynamic living properties of breast milk, and it is based on cow's milk protein, which is specific to the needs of calves. Human milk promotes brain development in babies and also contains vital immuno-globulins that strengthen your baby's immune system for life, helping to protect against disease. If circumstances allow—

- Let your baby nurse as long as he or she likes. Don't watch the clock. Plumpness is normal in a breastfed baby and is shed when the baby becomes mobile.
- Let your baby nurse as often as he or she likes. Feeding patterns vary. Your baby may nurse almost continuously in the late afternoons and less in the mornings, or the other way around.
- Let your baby lead the weaning. Breastfeeding can go on for as long as four or five years; this is completely normal for some mothers and their babies. There are no rules, but breastfeeding your baby for the first six months is most important. If you can continue for a year or longer, your baby will only benefit.

10 | Postpartum Exercises

IN THE FIRST WEEKS AFTER BIRTH YOUR MAIN CONCERN will be getting to know and taking care of your baby. You will need plenty of rest and a very nutritious diet, and you probably won't have much time or inclination for formal exercising. The many hours you will spend breastfeeding your baby are a perfect opportunity to rest, relax, and put your deep breathing into practice (see page 47). However, a few exercises are essential in helping your figure to return to its pre-pregnant state in the coming months. You will find a short exercise program is also an invaluable way to stay relaxed and to combat tiredness or lack of energy, which are so common in early motherhood.

The essential exercise program that follows has been designed to be followed in sequence, each exercise gradually strengthening the body in readiness for the next. The exercises begin the first day after birth and gradually build up to a program for the first six months. Although one week has been allocated for each sequence, it doesn't matter if it takes you 10 days or longer until you are ready to progress. It is important to follow your own rhythm and to fit exercising around the time spent with your baby, which should naturally be your first priority.

The postpartum exercise program concentrates on the following areas:

- Toning and firming the pelvic floor muscles and helping the uterus return to normal.
- Strengthening the lower back, which carries so much additional weight in pregnancy.
- Toning the abdominal muscles to restore their strength and elasticity.
- Releasing tension in the shoulders and neck—areas that are under stress from the many hours spent carrying your baby.
- Improving circulation to the breasts, maintaining tone in the muscles that support them, and maintaining good posture.
- Maintaining the increased flexibility and mobility of the joints that you achieved in pregnancy, while promoting the tightening of the ligaments.
- Lightening the pelvic area, and helping the return to normal curvature of the spine.
- Reducing fatigue and stimulating good energy flow and circulation.
- Relaxation.

Swimming and walking are excellent in combination with the exercise program, and they are enjoyable for your baby, too!

Never diet while you are breastfeeding. Your figure will slim down naturally if you maintain a sensible, well-balanced diet and exercise well.

You will find that many of the postpartum exercises recommended as follows are already old friends from the pregnancy program.

Week 1

1. On the first day or two after birth, lie on your belly in bed and tighten and release your pelvic floor muscles two or three times; then rest (see page 84). Do this several times a day. When the milk comes in and your breasts are tender, you may be more comfortable if you place a pillow under your ribs or only do the exercise lying on your back with knees bent (step 3).

2. Lie on your back on the floor in the basic reclining position (see page 86), with your hands on your belly and knees bent. Breathe deeply as before, but concentrate on tightening the abdominal muscles and drawing them down towards your spine when you exhale, releasing them when you inhale. Repeat up to 10 times.

3. In the same position, contract, hold, and release your pelvic floor muscles 10 times.

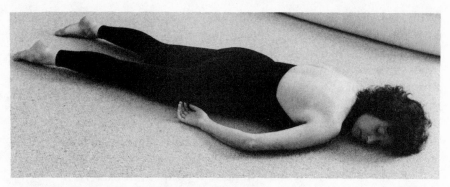

Position for the pelvic floor exercise after birth

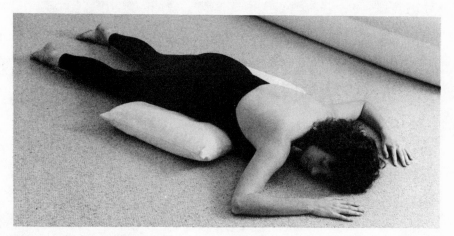

If your breasts are tender, try this.

4. After a postpartum check for separation of the recti (abdominal) muscles, begin the abdominal toner exercise (see page 63), but keep your feet on the floor. Build up to repeating 10 times. (See Elizabeth Noble's *Essential Exercises for the Childbearing Year* for information on testing for and correcting separation of the recti muscles.)

5. In the same position, do the pelvic lift (see page 86) and the lower back release (see page 88), to strengthen your spine.

6. Lie flat on your back with your legs and arms spread comfortably apart. Place a pillow under your knees, if you like. Tuck your chin in to relax the back of your neck, and close your eyes. Breathe deeply in and out through your nose, feeling the movement of the breath in your belly.

With each exhalation, relax each part of your body in turn, remembering to keep your jaw and eyes relaxed. Feel the way the back of your body contacts the floor. Let go of tension with each out-breath, so that your body sinks with gravity as you relax more and more deeply. Remain in this position for at least 10 minutes, pulling a blanket over yourself (keep one handy) if you are cold.

Known in yoga as the "corpse pose," this total relaxation should be practiced daily for 10 to 20 minutes, always at the end of your exercise session or on its own. It can be as relaxing as a few hours of sleep, and is therefore probably the most important postpartum exercise.

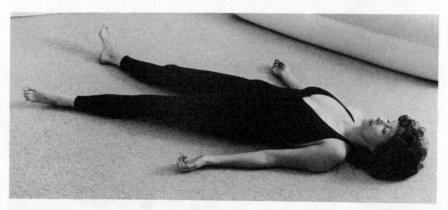

Total relaxation

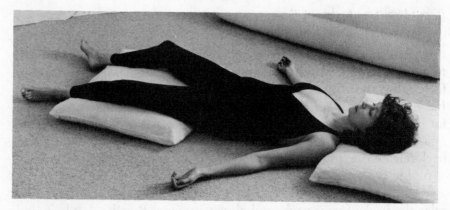

To increase your comfort while relaxing, try placing a pillow under your head and another under your knees.

Week 2

7. Add the tailor pose (see page 49).
8. Add the pelvic lift in the kneeling position (see page 58).

Week 3

9. Add kneeling with knees wide apart (see page 55).
10. Add the spinal twist (see page 58).

Weeks 4 to 6

11. Add the whole of exercise sequence VI, the shoulder release (see page 76).

Week 7 to 6 Months

12. Add legs apart on the wall (see page 65, steps 1 to 3).
13. Add the shoulder stand. *(Caution: Begin this exercise only after all bleeding from the uterus has ceased. Also, when doing this exercise do not turn your head to the side. If your baby calls, come down and out of the position.)*

Lie on your back with your buttocks close to the wall, in the same position as in "legs apart on the wall." Bend your knees, and place your feet together. Relax your shoulders, and place your arms by your sides with the palms down. Tuck in your chin to relax and lengthen the back of your neck (*a*). Breathe deeply into your belly, and relax all of your spine, especially your lower back, neck, and shoulders, onto the floor.

Tuck your elbows close into your sides, and drop them down onto the floor as you exhale. Then, keeping them in position, press your feet into the wall and lift your body up, supporting your upper back with your hands behind your ribs. Keep your neck and shoulders relaxed, and lift only as far as you can without strain. Straighten your legs, keeping your feet on the wall and your elbows down (*b*). At first your pelvis will feel very heavy, and you will have difficulty placing your hands on your upper

Shoulder stand

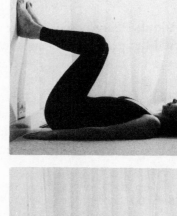

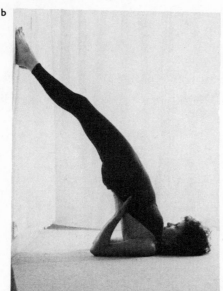

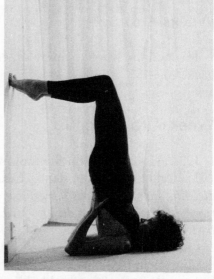

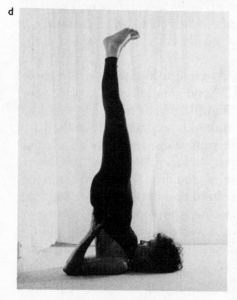

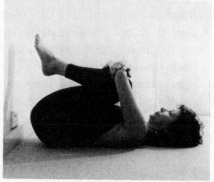

back, but with regular practice your neck will relax and your pelvis will become lighter. Concentrate on dropping your elbows as you exhale. Hold for a second, and then come down slowly on an exhalation. Hug your knees (*e*) to relax your lower back before coming up.

When this becomes easier, do the pelvic floor exercise before coming down: draw the pelvic floor down towards your navel when you contract, hold for a second, and then release; do this 10 times.

When straightening your legs with your feet against the wall becomes easy, bend your knees, and press the wall with your feet to bring your pelvis above your shoulders, so your trunk forms a 90-degree angle with the floor (*c*). Make sure your elbows are well tucked in. Place your hands behind your ribs, and drop your elbows as you exhale. Hold, and contract and release your pelvic floor 10 times. Then relax your spine onto the floor gently, and hug your knees (*e*) before coming up.

When achieving a 90-degree angle with your feet against the wall becomes easy (usually only after several weeks), try straightening your legs to find your balance. Your weight should be supported by your elbows and upper arms while your body forms a 90-degree angle to the floor (*d*). Contract and release your pelvic floor 10 times in this position. To come down, place your feet on the wall, and drop your spine gently from the neck towards the tailbone. Hug your knees (*e*) before coming up.

This exercise brings lightness to the pelvic area and aids recovery of the pelvic floor and uterus. After the first few weeks, the pelvic floor exercise should always be practiced in this position; done regularly, this can cure a prolapsed uterus and will reduce varicose veins, hemorrhoids, and vulval varicosities. The shoulder stand also releases tension in the upper back, neck, and shoulders, and benefits the endocrine system, helping you to regain hormonal balance after birth.

You can complete most of these essential exercises, except for total relaxation, in about 10 minutes. If you find you have time for only a few exercises, start with the legs apart on the wall, then do the tailor pose, the abdominal toner, and the shoulder stand.

As time and inclination allow, add the following to your exercise program: sitting with legs wide apart (see page 53); exercise sequence V, standing positions (page 68); the dog pose (page 80); and exercise sequence VIII, spinal release (page 86), omitting exercise E. Always end with total relaxation (page 92). In the months to come you will be ready to continue with more advanced yoga.

Emergency Birth:
For the Partner

If you are alone with a woman who is about to give birth and are unable to reach a midwife or doctor—

- Try to stay calm. Take a few deep breaths, with good, long out-breaths. *Surprise births are usually completely straightforward.* All you need to do is concentrate really well on what is happening.
- Comfort the mother and, if there is time, reassure her by holding her for a minute or two. Suggest that she get into the all-fours position (page 60) or the knee-chest position (page 131) while you get everything ready. This will help to slow down the contractions a little and will help her to feel more calm and in control. Give her a large cushion, if there is one.
- Get some clean towels, sheets, and a blanket, if possible, to cover the mother and the baby, and also a towel or receiving blanket to wrap the baby in.
- Close all windows, and try to warm the room, as the mother and baby will need to be kept very warm.
- If there is time, bring a kettle of water to a boil, then switch off the heat. Wash your hands really well. Get a glass of water, a bowl, and a roll of toilet paper or some absorbent cotton.
- Go back to the mother; massage her lower back gently and calmly. Give her sips of water and plenty of reassurance. Place a clean sheet, towel, or newspaper

underneath her, and have some more handy. Have a clean towel or blanket nearby to wrap the baby in. Place the towel or blanket near a heater to warm.

- Once you can give the mother your undivided attention, she can squat against a cushion or beanbag chair, if she prefers squatting to the all-fours position. Any position she chooses will be all right.

- All you have to do is concentrate and watch carefully for the appearance of the baby—your instincts will do the rest.

- Allow nature to take its course. Encourage the mother to take her time, to open up, and to give way to what is happening inside her. If she panics, breathe deeply with her, concentrating on the out-breath. Suggest that she breathe the baby out rather than push forcefully. Remind her to relax and slow down.

- If she is nauseated or vomits, don't worry. This is just a normal part of the expulsive reflex.

- If any feces come out of the mother's anus, wipe it clean with the toilet paper or cotton—away from the vagina.

- As the baby's head emerges, support it very gently in one hand.

- The baby may come out in one contraction, or else over several. Receive the baby without pulling. Allow the mother's uterus to do all the work; just let the baby emerge into your hands. Allow the head to hang down a little, as this will help the shoulders to come out.

- If the cord is around the baby's neck, as is quite common, simply place the baby down gently on its belly on a soft towel on the floor or bed. Then calmly free the cord from the baby's neck, unraveling it if necessary.

- If the mother is squatting, hold the baby face down between her feet for half a minute or so to drain the fluids, and then let the mother pick him or her up in her arms.

- If the mother is on all fours, hold the baby face down for a moment, and then pass the baby to the mother through her legs.

- The mother should sit upright with her baby. If a lot of fluid has come out of her, she can move over to a clean sheet or towel.

- Keep both the mother and baby warm with blanket, towel, coats, or whatever you have on hand. The top of the baby's head should be covered, too.

- Sit down and enjoy a few peaceful moments with mother and baby. Encourage the mother to put her baby to the breast, as this will stimulate the uterus to contract.

- Telephone for a midwife or doctor to come around.

- If the placenta comes out between the mother's legs, place it in a bowl. Don't cut the cord. It will stop pulsating and clamp itself spontaneously.

- After the placenta is out, the uterus should contract to the size and firmness of a grapefruit. If it doesn't, you or the mother should massage her belly firmly to stimulate the uterus to contract.

- If you have some, give the mother some arnica 30x or Bach rescue remedy (see page 197) and perhaps a cup of tea with sugar or honey.
- Use the previously boiled and cooled water from the kettle to wash the mother's genital area, or, better, let her squat over a bowl of warm water and do it herself. Then give her a sanitary napkin or clean towel to place between her legs and a pair of clean underpants.
- Don't leave the mother alone in the house.

If the birth takes place in a taxi or some other unusual place, your priorities should be to stay relaxed, reassure the mother, catch the baby, and make sure they are both warm before seeking help.

References

Chapter I

1. A. Prentice and T. Lind, "Fetal Heartrate Monitoring during Labour—Too Frequent Intervention, Too Little Benefit?" *Lancet* 2, no. 8572 (December 1987):1375–77.

2. Diana Korte and Roberta Scaer, *A Good Birth, a Safe Birth: Choosing and Having the Childbirth Experience You Want*, rev. ed. (Boston: Harvard Common Press, 1992).

3. Doris Haire, "Drugs in Labor," *Childbirth Educator*, Spring 1987.

4. W. Bowes et al., "The Side Effects of Obstetrical Medication on Fetus and Infant," *Monographs of the Society for Research in Child Development* 35, no. 137 (June 1970); T. Berry Brazelton, "Effect of Maternal Medications on the Neonate and His Behavior," *Journal of Pediatrics* 58:513–18; D. Rosenblatt, "The Influence of Maternal Analgesia on Neonatal Behaviour," *Journal of Obstetrics and Gynaecology of the British Commonwealth* 88 (April 1981):398–406; R. Kron, "Newborn Sucking Behavior Affected by Obstetric Sedation," *Journal of Pediatrics* 37:1012–16.

5. D. Rosenblatt, "The Influence of Maternal Analgesia on Neonatal Behaviour."

6. I. J. Hoult, A. H. MacLennon, and L. E. S. Carrie, "Lumbar Epidural

Analgesia in Labour: Relation to Fetal Malposition and Instrumental Delivery," *British Medical Journal* 1, no. 6052 (January 1977):14–16.

7. D. Rosenblatt, "The Influence of Maternal Analgesia on Neonatal Behaviour."

8. Doris Haire, "The Cultural Warping of Childbirth," *Childbirth Educator,* Spring 1987.

9. P. Hubinot et al., "Effects of Vacuum Extractor and Obstetrical Forceps on the Foetus and Newborn—a Comparison," World Congress on Gynaecology and Obstetrics, Sydney, Australia, 1967.

10. D. Rosenblatt, "Epidural Buvacaine," *Journal of Obstetrics and Gynaecology of the British Commonwealth* 88 (April 1981):407–17; "Regionals Can Prolong Labor," *Medical World News,* 15 October 1971, p. 41; N. Potter and R. D. Macdonald, "Obstetric Consequences of Epidural Analgesia on Nulliparous Patients," *Lancet* 1, no. 7708 (May 1971):1031–34; L. Hellman and J. Pritchard, *Williams Obstetrics,* 14th ed. (NY: Appleton-Century-Crofts, 1971).

11. Haire, Doris, "Drugs in Labor."

12. R. W. Taylor and M. Taylor, "Misuse of Oxytocin in Labour," *Lancet* 1, no. 8581 (February 1988):352; I. Chalmers, H. Campbell, and A. Turnbull, "Use of Oxytocin and Incidence of Neonatal Jaundice," *British Medical Journal* 2:116.

13. P. Steer et al., *Journal of Obstetrics and Gynaecology of the British Commonwealth* 92 (November 1985):1120–1126; H. Fields, "Induction of Labour: Methods, Hazards, Complications and Contraindications," *Hospital Topics,* December 1968:63–68; H. Fields, "Complications of Elective Induction," *Obstetrics and Gynaecology* 15:476–80; W. A. Liston and A. J. Campbell, "Dangers of Oxytocin Induced Labour to the Fetus," *British Medical Journal* 3, no. 5931 (September 1974):606–7.

14. P. M. Dunn, "François Mauriceau (1637–1709) and Maternal Posture for Parturition," *MIDIRS Midwifery Digest* 1, no. 2 (June 1991):71.

15. G. J. Englemann, *Labor Among Primitive Peoples* (Cleveland: Burke, 1882).

16. J. G. B. Russell, "Moulding of the Pelvic Outlet," *Journal of Obstetrics and Gynaecology of the British Commonwealth* 76 (1969):817–20.

17. D. B. Scott and N. G. Kerr, "Inferior Vena Caval Pressure in Late Pregnancy," *Journal of Obstetrics and Gynaecology of the British Commonwealth* 70 (1963):1044–1049.

18. A. M. Flynn et al., "Ambulation in Labour," *British Medical Journal,* August 1978:591–93.

19. R. Caldeyro-Barcia, "The Influence of Maternal Position on Time of Spontaneous Rupture of the Membranes, Progress of Labour and Fetal Head Compression," *Birth and the Family Journal* 6, no. 1 (Spring 1979):7–15; I. N.

Mitre, "The Influence of Maternal Position on Duration of the Active Phase of Labour," *International Journal of Gynaecology and Obstetrics* 12, no. 5 (September 1984):181–83; Y. C. Liu, "Effects of an Upright Position during Labor," *American Journal of Nursing* 74 (1974):2202–5; Y. C. Liu, "Position during Labor and Delivery: History and Perspective," *Journal of Nurse-Midwifery* 24 (1979):23–26.

20. P. M. Dunn, "Posture in Labour," *Lancet* 1, no. 8062 (March 1978):492–97, 1978.

21. M. C. Botha, "The Management of the Umbilical Cord in Labour," *South African Journal of Obstetrics and Gynaecology* 6, no. 2:30–33, 1968.

22. A. Blankfield, "The Optimum Position for Childbirth," *Medical Journal of Australia* 2 (1965):666–68; F. H. Howard, "Delivery in the Physiologic Position," *Obstetrics and Gynaecology* 11 (1958):318–22; I. Gritsivk, "Position in Labour," *Obstetrics-Gynaecology Observer*, September 1968; N. Newton and M. Newton, "The Propped Position for the Second Stage of Labour," *Obstetrics and Gynaecology* 15 (1960):28–34.

23. Michel Odent, "Towards Less Mechanized Childbirth: The Pithiviers Experience," in *Advances in International Maternal and Child Health* 5, ed. D. B. Jelliffe and E. F. P. Jelliffe (Oxford: Clarendon Press, 1985).

24. In *Planned Home Birth in Industrialized Countries*, a report Odent wrote for the World Health Organization (Copenhagen: World Health Organization, 1991), he stated: "The priority must be to challenge the universal propaganda that home birth is dangerous. . . . The best means by which to challenge the current beliefs are the statistics from the Netherlands. . . . The Netherlands is the only industrialized country where one-third of all births happen at home. The Netherlands is also the only country where they can reconcile a perinatal mortality rate lower than 10 per 1,000, a maternal mortality rate lower than 1 per 10,000, and a rate of caesarean section of around 6%."

25. At this writing the Active Birth Unit at the Garden Hospital is facing closure. It will have moved to different premises in February 1992. For the new address, contact the Active Birth Centre (see "Resources").

Chapter 6

1. *MIDIRS Database on Position and Ambulation in Labour* (Bristol, England: Midwives Information and Resource Service).

2. Michel Odent, "The Fetus Ejection Reflex," *Birth* 14 (June 1987); N. Newton, "The Fetus Ejection Reflex Revisited," *Birth* 14 (June 1987).

3. N. Newton, D. Foshee, and M. Newton, "Experimental Inhibition of Labour through Environmental Disturbance," *Obstetrics and Gynaecology* 67 (1966):371–77.

Chapter 7

1. A. Prentice and T. Lind, "Fetal Heartrate Monitoring during Labor—Too Frequent Intervention, Too Little Benefit?"
2. Sheila Kitzinger, ed., *Episiotomy—Physical and Emotional Aspects* (London: National Childbirth Trust, 1981), p. 6.
3. Penny Simkin, *The Birth Partner* (Boston: Harvard Common Press, 1989), p. 172.

Chapter 8

1. Eric Sidenbladh, *Water Babies* (London: Adam & Charles Black, 1983); Karil Daniels, *The Water Baby Information Book* (San Francisco: Point of View Productions, 1990).
2. Michel Odent, "Birth under Water," *Lancet* 2, no. 8355/8356 (December 1983):1476–77.
3. Michel Odent, *Birth Reborn* (New York: Pantheon, 1984).
4. Michel Odent, "Birth under Water."
5. International contacts for water birth and a video entitled *Water Baby—Experiences of Water Birth* can be obtained from Karil Daniels of Point of View Productions (see "Resources").
6. Michel Odent, "Birth under Water."
7. M. Rosenthal, "Water Birth: An American Experience," in *The Water Baby Information Book*, ed. Karil Daniels.
8. Igor Tjarkovsky maintains that the partner's entering the pool is unlikely to increase the risk of infection if the partner and mother normally share the same bacteriological environment.

Chapter 9

1. Michel Odent, *Primal Health* (London: Century Hutchinson, 1986).
2. Sally Inch, *Birthrights: A Parents' Guide to Modern Childbirth*, 2nd ed. (London: Green Print Merlin Press, 1989).

Recommended Reading

Exercise

Noble, Elizabeth. *Essential Exercises for the Childbearing Year*, 3rd ed. Boston: Houghton Mifflin, 1988.

Olkin, Sylvia Klein. *Positive Pregnancy Fitness: A Guide to a More Comfortable Pregnancy and Easier Birth through Exercise and Relaxation*. Wayne, N.J.: Avery Publishing Group, 1987.

Pregnancy and Birth

Balaskas, Janet. *Natural Pregnancy: A Practical Holistic Guide to Wellbeing from Conception to Birth*. New York: Interlink, 1990.

Balaskas, Janet, and Yehudi Gordon. *The Encyclopedia of Pregnancy and Birth*. London: Macdonald Orbis, 1987. (Available from the Active Birth Centre or ICEA by mail-order; see "Resources.")

Baldwin, Rahima, and Terra Palmarini. *Pregnant Feelings*. Berkeley: Celestial Arts, 1986.

Brewer, Gail Sforza, and Tom Brewer. *What Every Pregnant Woman Should Know: The Truth about Diets and Drugs in Pregnancy*. New York: Penguin, 1985.

Brewer, Gail Sforza, and Janice Green. *Right from the Start: Meeting the Challenges of Mothering Your Unborn and Newborn Baby.* Emmaus, Penn.: Rodale, 1981.

Davis, Elizabeth. *Energetic Pregnancy.* Berkeley: Celestial Arts, 1988.

Kitzinger, Sheila. *The Complete Book of Pregnancy and Childbirth,* rev. ed. New York: Knopf, 1989.

Kitzinger, Sheila. *The Experience of Childbirth,* 5th ed. New York: Penguin, 1984.

Kitzinger, Sheila, and Penny Simkin, eds. *Episiotomy and the Second Stage of Labor,* 2nd ed. Seattle: Pennypress, 1986.

Leboyer, Frederick. *Birth without Violence.* New York: Knopf, 1975.

Noble, Elizabeth. *Childbirth with Insight.* Boston: Houghton Mifflin, 1983.

Odent, Michel. *Birth Reborn.* New York: Pantheon, 1986.

Panuthos, Claudia. *Transformation through Birth: A Woman's Guide.* South Hadley, Mass.: Bergin Garvey, 1984.

Peterson, Gayle. *Birthing Normally: A Personal Growth Approach to Childbirth,* 2nd rev. ed. Berkeley: Mindbody Press, 1984.

Peterson, Gayle, and Lewis Mehl. *Pregnancy as Healing.* Berkeley: Mindbody Press, 1984.

Simkin, Penny, Janet Whalley, and Ann Keppler. *Pregnancy, Childbirth, and the Newborn: A Complete Guide for Expectant Parents.* Deephaven, Minn.: Meadowbrook Press, 1984.

Home Birth and Midwifery

Arms, Suzanne. *Immaculate Deception: A New Look at Women and Childbirth.* South Hadley, Mass.: Bergin & Garvey, 1984.

Baldwin, Rahima. *Special Delivery: The Complete Guide to Informed Birth.* Berkeley: Celestial Arts, 1986.

Davis, Elizabeth. *Heart and Hands: A Midwife's Guide to Pregnancy and Birth.* Berkeley: Celestial Arts, 1987.

Gaskin, Ina May. *Spiritual Midwifery,* 3rd ed. Summertown, Tenn.: Book Publishing Co., 1990.

Haire, Doris. *The Cultural Warping of Childbirth.* Seattle: ICEA Supplies Center, 1972.

Cesarean Birth

Cohen, Nancy Wainer, and Lois J. Estner. *Silent Knife: Cesarean Prevention and Vaginal Birth after Cesarean.* South Hadley, Mass.: Bergin & Garvey, 1983.

Partners

Simkin, Penny. *The Birth Partner: Everything You Need to Know to Help a Woman through Childbirth.* Boston: Harvard Common Press, 1989.

Water Birth

Daniels, Karil, ed. *The Water Baby Information Book.* San Francisco: Point of View Productions, 1990.

Balaskas, Janet, and Yehudi Gordon. *Water Birth.* London: Thorsons, 1990. (Available by mail-order from the Active Birth Centre or ICEA; see "Resources.")

Breastfeeding

Huggins, Kathleen. *The Nursing Mother's Companion*, rev. ed. Boston: Harvard Common Press, 1990.

Kitzinger, Sheila. *The Experience of Breastfeeding*, rev. ed. Penguin, 1985.

La Leche League International. *The Womanly Art of Breastfeeding*, 4th ed. Franklin Park, Ill.: La Leche League International, 1987.

Renfrew, Mary, Chloe Fisher, and Suzanne Arms. *Bestfeeding: Getting Breastfeeding Right for You.* Berkeley: Celestial Arts, 1990.

Touch and Massage

Montagu, Ashley. *Touching: The Human Significance of the Skin*, 3rd ed. New York: Harper and Row, 1986.

Teeguarden, Iona. *The Joy of Feeling: Body-Mind Acupressure.* Tokyo and New York: Japan Publications, 1987.

Resources

Active Birth Centre
25 Bickerton Road
London N19 5JT
United Kingdom

Directed by Janet Balaskas and her husband, Keith Brainin, this is the international center for the Active Birth Movement. The center provides training for prospective active birth teachers all over the world, advice on active birth, and a mail-order catalog. Included in the catalog are two video tapes by Janet Balaskas—*Preparing for Active Birth* and *Active Birth and Water Birth at Home and in Hospital*—as well as an audio cassette and booklet on yoga for pregnancy. Also available, for rental or purchase, are Aqua Birth Pools, which were designed by Keith Brainin with the help of Michel Odent. The pools are available in both installed and portable models.

American College of Nurse-Midwives
818 Connecticut Avenue, NW
Suite 900
Washington, DC 20006
202-728-9860
e-mail: info@acnm.org
web site: www.midwife.org

This organization, which establishes and maintains standards for the practice of midwifery, can refer you to certified nurse-midwives practicing in your area.

American College of Obstetricians and Gynecologists
Resource Center
409 Twelfth Street, SW
Washington, DC 20024
202-638-5577
web site: www.acog.com

Besides setting national standards in obstetrical education and practice, this organization offers free pamphlets on many topics concerning pregnancy and birth.

American Foundation for Maternal and Child Health
439 East 51st Street
New York, New York 10022
212-759-5510
e-mail: aims@comet.net

This foundation, headed by Doris Haire, provides scientific information on potentially harmful obstetrical practices.

ASPO/Lamaze
1200 Nineteenth Street, NW
Suite 300
Washington, DC 20036
800-368-4404 or 202-857-1128
e-mail: aspo@sba.com
web site: www.lamaze-childbirth.com

The oldest childbirth education program in America, ASPO/Lamaze provides referrals to local certified Lamaze instructors. Videos, books, and pamphlets on pregnancy and labor are also available by mail order.

Cesarean/Support, Education and Concern (C/SEC, Inc.)
22 Forest Road
Framingham, Massachusetts 01701
508-877-8266

C/SEC provides emotional support to women who have given birth by cesarean. The organization publishes booklets on cesarean childbirth, cesarean prevention, and VBAC.

Childbirth Graphics, a division of WRS Group, Inc.
P.O. Box 21207
Waco, Texas 76702
800-299-3366 x287
e-mail: sales@wrsgroup.com

This mail-order company offers books, pamphlets, and tapes on birth and parenting.

Homeopathic Associations
International Foundation
for Homeopathy
P.O. Box 7
Edmonds, Washington 98020
206-776-4147
e-mail: ifh@nwlink.com

National Center for Homeopathy
801 North Fairfax Street
Suite 306
Alexandria, Virginia 22314
703-548-7790
e-mail: nchinfo@igc.apc.org
web site: www.homeopathic.org

Homeopathic Suppliers
Ehrhart and Karl, Ltd.
30 South Wacker Drive
Suite 1620
Chicago, Illinois 60606
800-607-7447

Homeopathic Educational Services
2124 Kittredge Street
Berkeley, California 947074
510-649-0294
e-mail: mail@homeopathic.com
web site: www.homeopathic.com

Luyties Pharmacal Company
P.O. Box 8080
St. Louis, Missouri 63156
314-533-9600

Standard Homeopathic Company
154 West 131st Street
Los Angeles, California 90061
800-624-9659 or 213-321-4284

Washington Homeopathic Products
4914 Del Ray Avenue
Bethesda, Maryland 20814
301-656-1695

If you cannot find homeopathic medicines in a local pharmacy or health-food store, you can obtain them by mail-order from any of these companies.

Informed Home Birth/Informed Birth and Parenting Bookstore
P.O. Box 3675
Ann Arbor, Michigan 48106
313-662-6857

This organization offers a mail-order catalog of books on home birth and early childhood education.

International Association of Parents and Professionals for Safe Alternatives in Childbirth (NAPSAC, International)
Route 1, Box 646
Marble Hill, Missouri 63764
573-238-2010
e-mail: stewartdl@compuserve.com

An umbrella organization for the alternative birth movement, NAPSAC offers a quarterly newsletter, a mail-order book service, and an international directory of alternative birth services.

International Cesarean Awareness Network (ICAN)
1304 Kingsdale Avenue
Redondo Beach, California 90278
310-542-6400
e-mail: ICANinc@aol.com
web site: www.childbirth.org/section/ican

This organization offers a newsletter, conferences, and nationwide support groups for cesarean prevention and vaginal birth after cesarean.

International Childbirth Education Association (ICEA)
P.O. Box 20048
Minneapolis, Minnesota 55420
612-854-8660
e-mail: info@icea.org
web site: www.icea.org

ICEA member groups offer classes, a journal, and a catalog of books and pamphlets on childbirth and family-centered maternity care. The catalog includes other books by Janet Balaskas.

La Leche League International
1400 North Meacham Road
Schaumburg, Illinois 60173
800-LA-LECHE

Call between 9:00 A.M. and 3:00 P.M. CST for breastfeeding help or a referral to a local La Leche breastfeeding support group.

Maternity Center Association
48 East 92nd Street
New York, New York 10128
212-777-5000

In addition to running a birth center and conducting classes and conferences, the Center publishes many booklets on childbirth. Send for a complete list.

Midwives Alliance of North America (MANA)
P.O. Box 175
Newton, Kansas 67114
316-283-4543
e-mail: manainfo@aol.com
web site: www.mana.org

MANA can provide you information on midwifery and referrals to midwives in your area.

Mothering Magazine
P.O. Box 1690
Santa Fe, New Mexico 87504
800-984-8116 or 505-984-8116
e-mail: mother@ni.net

This quarterly magazine of alternative advice for parents also offers packets of reprints on lay midwifery, circumcision, and vaccination.

National Women's Health Network
514 Tenth Street, NW
Suite 400
Washington, DC 20004
202-347-1140

The Network monitors federal policies that affect women's health, especially in the areas of reproductive rights and environmental and occupational health. A newsletter and other publications are available.

Nursing Mothers Counsel
P.O. Box 50063
Palo Alto, California 94303
415-591-6688

Nursing Mothers Counsel offers breastfeeding support through chapters in various cities in California and in Denver, Fort Wayne, and Atlanta. Call for a local number.

Point of View Productions
2477 Folsom Street
San Francisco, California 94110
415-821-0435
web site: www.well.com/user/karil

Karil Daniels provides information on water birth. Her products include the annually updated *Water Baby Information Book*, a video tape (available in all formats), an audio tape, and a resource list.

Vaginal Birth after Cesarean (VBAC)
10 Great Plain Terrace
Needham, Massachusetts 02192
617-449-2490

Nancy Wainer Cohen, author of *Silent Knife*, provides counseling and workshops on vaginal birth after cesarean section.

Water Birth International, a project of Global Maternal/Child Health Association
P.O. Box 1400
Wilsonville, Oregon 97070
503-682-3600
e-mail: waterbirth@aol.com
web site: www.geocities.com/hotsprings/2840

Directed by Barbara Harper, this organization provides information on natural birth, including birth in water, and sells books and video tapes by mail-order. Water Birth International also rents and sells portable, inflatable birthing tubs, which can be shipped anywhere in the United States.

Index